FALSE PREMISES

FALSE PROMISES

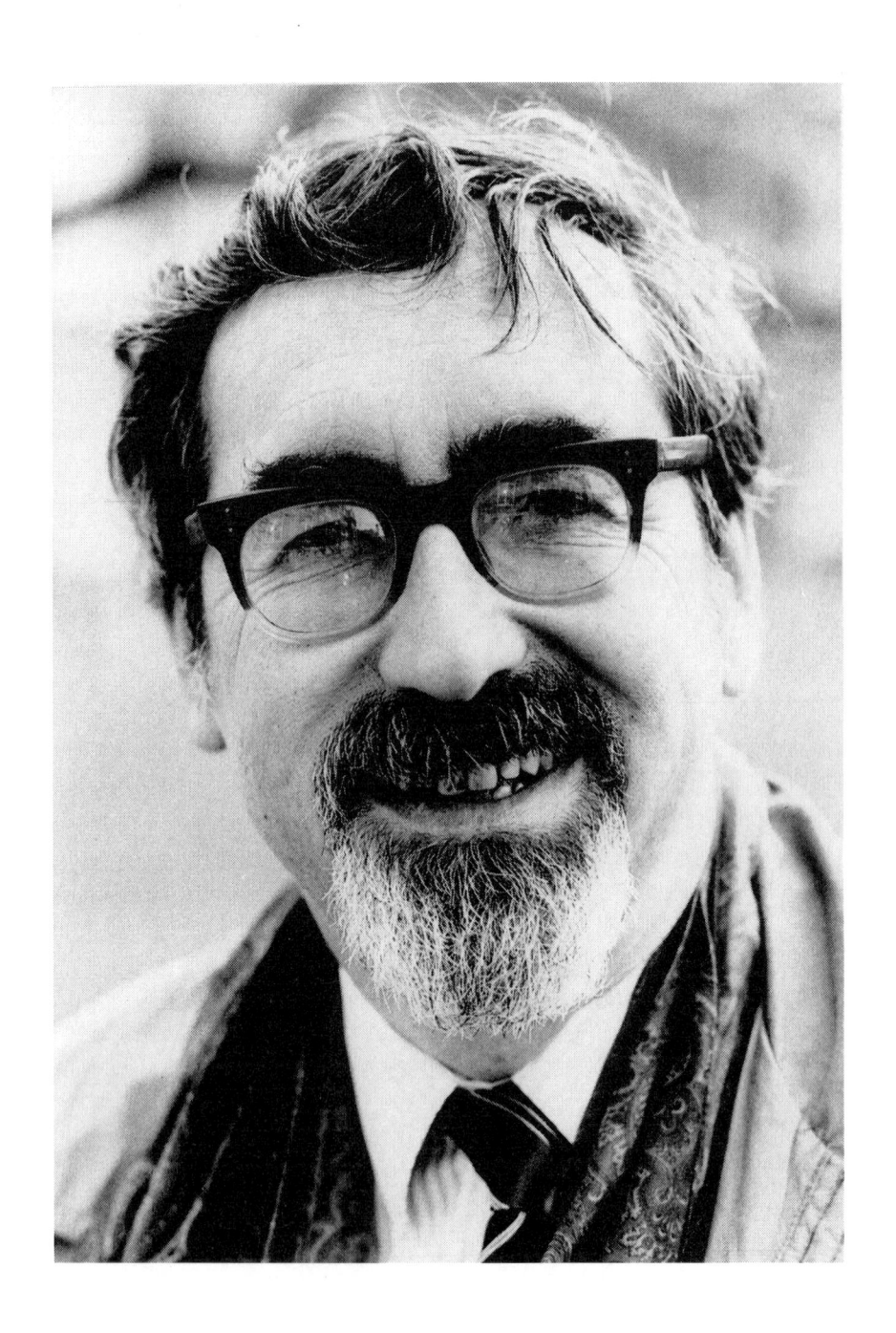

FALSE PREMISES

FALSE PROMISES

Selected writings of

PETR SKRABANEK

With an introduction by
Professor George Davey Smith

Tarragon Press
for the Skrabanek Foundation

This collection first published May 2000

ISBN 1 870781 11 2

Typeset in 10 pt Bookman by Tarragon Press, Whithorn
Printed by Antony Rowe Ltd, Chippenham

CONTENTS

Petr Skrabanek 1940-1994		vii
Petr Skrabanek and the Limits of Epidemiology		xi
George Davey Smith		

Selected Papers of Petr Skrabanek

1	In Defence of Destructive Criticism	1
2	False Premises and False Promises of Breast Cancer Screening	11
3	Acupuncture: Past, Present and Future	29
4	Convulsive Therapy — a Critical Appraisal of its Origins and Value	53
5	From Language to Lesion	79
6	Scepticism, Irrationalism and pseudoscience	106
7	Cervical Cancer in Nuns and Prostitutes: A Plea for Scientific Continence	120
8	Provision for Research with Animals	132
9	Nonsensus Consensus	139
10	Why is preventive medicine exempted from ethical constraints ?	143
11	Risk-Factor Epidemiology: Science or Non-science ?	153
12	Smoking and Society	164
13	The Poverty of Epidemiology	178
14	The Emptiness of the Black Box	183
15	Irish traditional medicine: the foxglove ordeal and other folk 'cures'	189
16	A subversive man	204

PETR SKRABANEK 1940-1994

Petr was born in Nachod in Bohemia in 1940 and it was there he spent his childhood. Nachod is a provincial town but one with a lively cultural tradition. When still at school he developed a passionate interest in chemistry and in due course entered Charles University to read natural sciences.

While still a student he worked as an honorary research assistant at the Institute for Toxicology and Forensic Medicine and at the remarkably young age of twenty two was appointed head of the Toxicology Department at the Institute for Forensic Medicine, Purkyne University in Brno. At this time he also became a regular contributor to Chemical Abstracts and to *Vesmir* (Cosmos), a leading Czechoslovakian natural science journal.

In 1963, aged twenty three, he began his medical studies at Purkyne University. In 1967, as an outstanding student, he was selected to spend time abroad and spent a month at University College Galway. He fell in love with Ireland and a year later returned to spend a month in a Dublin teaching hospital. This was the time of the Prague Spring and his wife Vera was allowed to join him for a brief holiday. It was in the west of Ireland and while visiting Yeats' grave at Drumcliffe in Sligo that they heard the news of the Soviet invasion of Czechoslovakia. Despite the fact that their total assets were a small tent, two rucksacks and only indifferent English, their experience of totalitarianism was such that they decided to remain in Ireland. This extraordinarily brave decision meant that they were immediately cut off from both family and friends. However thanks to much kindness and support Petr was given a post in the Medical Council Laboratories in Dublin.

A year later he was admitted to the medical school of the Royal College of Surgeons in Ireland and qualified in 1970. From then until 1975 he worked as intern, senior house officer and finally registrar in neurology.

In 1975 he left clinical medicine to become Senior Research Fellow in the Endocrine Oncology Unit in the Mater Hospital. His work centred on the neurotransmitter Substance P on which he became a world authority. He also found time to complete his doctoral thesis on "Inappropriate production of hormonal peptides in neoplasia". During these years he began to publish on issues of more general concern. Some of these so impressed the editor that he became an occasional editorialist for 'The Lancet'.

In 1984 he joined the Department of Community Health in Trinity College, initially in a temporary capacity, aided by a grant from the Wellcome Foundation. It was then that he began to establish his reputation as cogent and fearless critic particularly in relation to preventive medicine. In 1986 he became tenured and was rapidly promoted from lecturer to senior lecturer and finally to associate professor. He was made a fellow of the College and, very unusually, a fellow of the Royal College of Physicians of Ireland.

All those who knew Petr were in awe of his formidable intellect and the depth and width of his learning. His second major reputation was as a Joycean scholar and every year he gave a series of seminars on *Finnegans Wake*. He was much in demand as a speaker and seminarist throughout Europe and America. He had a wide circle of friends from all over the world, in part a result of his habit of writing to those whose work he admired. A realist, a sceptic not a cynic, he had little hope that there would ever be a limit to human foolishness and viewed the future with some degree of pessimism. Pessimism which did not in any way diminish his pleasure in his friends, in pints and in conversation. Talking which was always illuminated by the richness of the sources upon which he could draw. He was both chess player and pianist: late at night he would play boogie-woogie and jazz with panache and only occasional inaccuracy. His capacity for productive work was almost incredible. He worked best in the evenings and night and would be busy typing into the small hours before retiring to take solace in Montaigne's essays. By the time of his death he had published over three hundred pieces and during his last illness finished his book 'The Death of

Humane Medicine" which was published posthumously.

For Petr the most important thing in life was his love for Vera and their daughters and it was good that he was able to die at home. Future generations will honour his learning, the elegance of his writing and the cogency of his criticism. Those who knew and loved him will treasure the privilege of having known such a remarkable man.

PETR SKRABANEK AND THE LIMITS OF EPIDEMIOLOGY

George Davey Smith

Epidemiology provides a good example of the dictum that the smaller and more specialised a particular field is, the more ferocious are the internal battles fought by the initiates. Over the past few years the "epidemiology wars"[1] have intensified considerably, in ways which, I am sure, would have entertained and engaged Petr Skrabanek's interest and elicited further contributions from him. There are several separate dimensions to critiques of current epidemiological practice, with diametrically opposed views being expressed on several key issues by different commentators. As is often the case, however, the various criticisms are sometimes linked in ways which suggest they are mutually reinforcing, when on occasion they point in different directions. The apparent crisis in epidemiology is, in fact, a series of crises — although most commentators have been particularly engaged with one aspect of epidemiology's malaise.

Why should problems within a small academic discipline — a subspecialty within preventive and social medicine, itself a minor part of the medical enterprise — be of interest to other than professionals earning their living within the field? Epidemiology certainly elicits emotional responses. In his recent pop-history *The rise and fall of modern medicine*[2], the medical journalist James Le Fanu went so far as to suggest that the solution to the fall of his title was to close all departments of epidemiology. If it would work this certainly sounds a cost-effective approach to problems within medicine (except to those of us who would be looking for alternative employment opportunities). Can epidemiology really be responsible for the current malaise in the medical enterprise? The suggestion that it might is certainly helped by the high profile epidemiology receives in the popular media. In Britain the broadsheet daily newspapers tend to pick one medical story out of the weekly medical journals which are published on a Friday. More often than not the highlighted story will be an epidemiological one — some aspect of daily life has been shown by epidemiologists to be bad for people. In the U.S. these stories seem to hit the T.V. screens more than in Britain, as the cartoon illustrates (Figure 1).

The failings of epidemiology that have been identified in recent critiques embrace most aspects of the epidemiological enterprise. First, the propensity of "risk factor epidemiology" to become the indiscriminate identification of particular aspects of daily life as dangerous to health — as reflected in the cartoons (Figures 1 and 2) — has been widely condemned. Second, critics censure the willingness of epidemiologists to accept "black box" associations between exposures and disease as serious contenders for causal relationships, with no understanding of biological mechanisms. Third, many preventive medicine campaigns — regarding diet, drinking, smoking, recreational drugs, forms of sexual behaviour, tanning, sloth, obesity — are seen to be driven more by moralism than by science. Epidemiology is, from this perspective, not value free, but a tool used to support predetermined goals. Fourth, epidemiology as it is currently practised is seen to be excessively concerned with individual risks and inadequately engaged with the social production of disease.

Unusually for a critic of epidemiology, Petr Skrabanek wrote and talked about all of these problems within the epidemiological enterprise, although he was particularly engaged with the first three. The present collection contains some of his writings on these issues, along with other pieces which display the extraordinary range of his interests and erudition. While some potential preface writers may have the same sweeping breadth of expertise as Petr, the present one does not, and therefore in this introductory essay (which is based on the third Skrabanek memorial lecture, given in Dublin on March 26th 1999) I will concentrate on Petr's writings on the problems which exist in the practice and use of epidemiology.

Risk factor epidemiology

A major component of Petr's attack on epidemiology relates to what he termed "risk-factorology". This is the practice of performing studies which relate a myriad of potential exposures to disease risk and

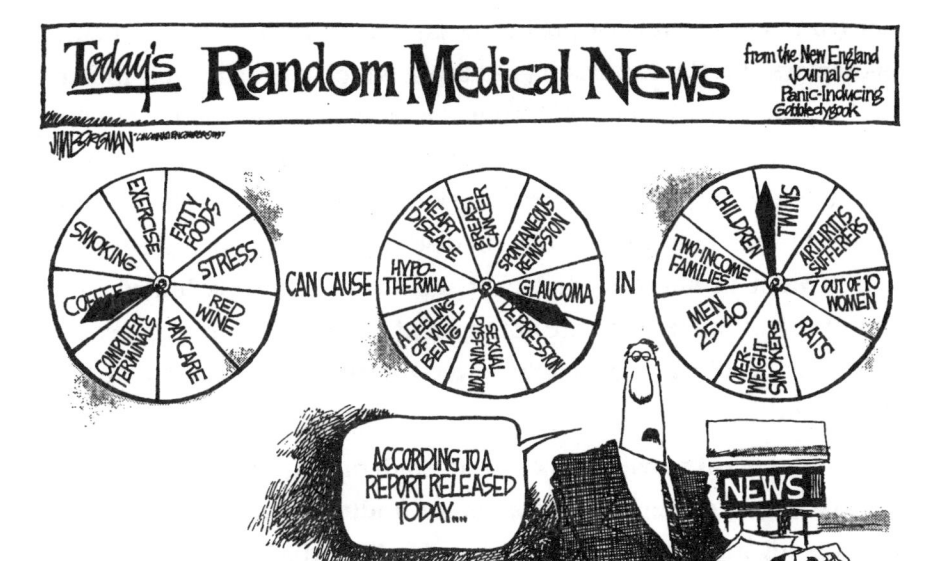

Figure 1

"DON'T EAT EGGS.... EAT MORE EGGS..... TOMATOES ARE GOOD FOR PROSTATES.... TAKE MORE VITAMINS... VITAMINS CAUSE CANCER.... STAY OUT OF THE SUN.... DON'T LIE AROUND INSIDE........ OH, AND CUT DOWN ON STRESS."

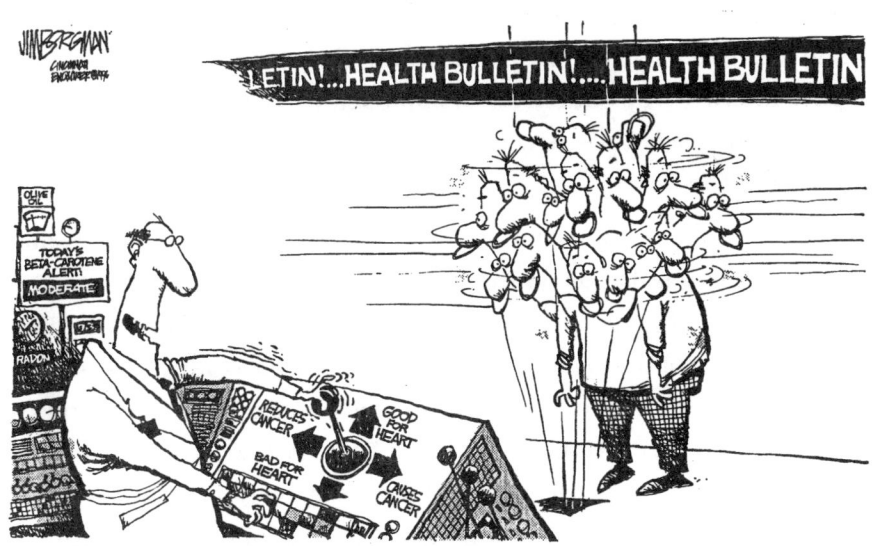

Figure 2

Reprinted with special permission of King Features Syndicate identifying those which are positively associated with disease as being "risk factors" for the condition (and those which are negatively linked as being protective factors). Although it is continuously pointed out (by the risk-factorologists among others) that association does not mean causation, the major reason for doing such studies — as Petr notes in chapter 11 — is to identify causes of disease. There is not a great deal of excitement in showing that cabbage consumption is linked to a lowered risk of cancer if it were not thought that by encouraging people to eat more cabbage you would lower the burden of cancer in the population.

A particular weakness of risk factor epidemiology is that different investigators often report contradictory findings from such studies. Petr gives several examples in chapters 11, 13 and 14, and others have systematically demonstrated the degree of disagreement that can be found in such studies[3]. As Petr points out, this apparent weakness of the method can be turned to an advantage, since once a positive association has been identified further positive studies are noteworthy (replication being the hallmark of science, perhaps a genuine cause is being identified ?) while negative findings may be controversial and thus of interest. The bottom line, it almost always seems, is that "more research is needed" — a conclusion comforting to epidemiologists working in the field.

Without previous positive associations having been reported, studies finding no association between a potential risk factor and a disease are unlikely to be of great interest. The published epidemiological literature certainly contains reports of more positive associations than null results — an example of "publication bias", whereby only apparently exciting findings reach the light of day. By this means alone a host of purely chance findings will be published, as by conventional reasoning examining 20 associations will find one "statistically significant at the p=0.05 level" result. If only the positive findings are published then their being the necessary outlying tail of the distribution of associations will not be noticed, and they may be mistaken for meaningful links between exposure and disease. Since many studies contain long questionnaires collecting information on hundreds of variables, and measure a wide range of potential outcomes, several false positive findings are virtually guaranteed. Petr emphasised the chance nature of apparent epidemiological "findings" in many places (chapters 11, 13 and 14).

The situation is probably worse than even this reasoning suggests. The percentage of apparent findings which are "false positives" will depend on the proportion of associations which are examined that, in the real world, are related. The table below represents the scenario in which the proportion of hypotheses tested in epidemiological studies which are real associations is 1 in 10.

Hypothetical test of 10,000 associations in epidemiological studies, with average power of 0.5 and a Type 1 error rate of 5%

(Adapted from Oakes[4])

	How the World is	
Decision	Null hypothesis true	Null hypothesis false
Accept null hypothesis	8550	500 Type 2 errors
Reject null hypothesis	450 Type 1 errors	500

We consider the situation where the power of studies which are carried out is 0.5, which means that there is a 50% chance of detecting real effects if they exist. This is reflected in the "null hypothesis false" column, where 50% of the time the null hypothesis (of no association) is rejected (i.e. it is assumed that there is a real effect). Imagine that 10,000 associations are examined and that 90% of the associations which are tested reflect hypotheses which are not valid (i.e. are cases when the null hypothesis should be accepted). At the conventional significance level of p=0.05, 450 out of 9,000 times the statistical test will have wrongly rejected the null hypothesis (which is referred to as a type 1 error), since 450 divided by 9,000 = 0.05. Thus, of the 950 cases where the null hypothesis is rejected, 500 times it is rejected correctly and 450 times it is rejected incorrectly. In other words 450/950 of the time — on nearly half of the occasions — apparently statistically significant findings are type 1 errors.[4] Remember that this example relates to a case where 1 in 10 associations exist in the real world. The actual situation is probably worse than this, since the nature of many epidemiological studies means that a great magnitude of potential associations can be examined, especially when each potential association can be looked at within many subgroups (men, women, the young, the elderly, those with existing disease, those without existing disease, those with high blood pressure, those with normal blood pressure, etc).

Petr made great play of the near-random nature of epidemiological associations which have been identified in the literature, and the above reasoning demonstrates why these may appear. These supposed "findings" do not reflect links in the outside world, they are constructed by the epidemiologist's methods of examining data and reporting results. A second set of associations can be uncovered which do exist in the real world, but may have a different meaning than is conventionally attached to them. To illustrate this I would like the reader to inspect Figure 3. This demonstrates the association between cigarette smoking and the risk of dying from 3 causes of death in a follow-up study of a third of a million men in the U.S. The vertical axis represents the relative risk of dying, with the baseline (relative risk = 1) being for non-smokers and a relative risk of 2 indicating twice the risk of dying for the group which experiences it. Thus for cause of death A the men who smoked 1-19 cigarettes per day (less than 1 pack per day) had 1.4 times

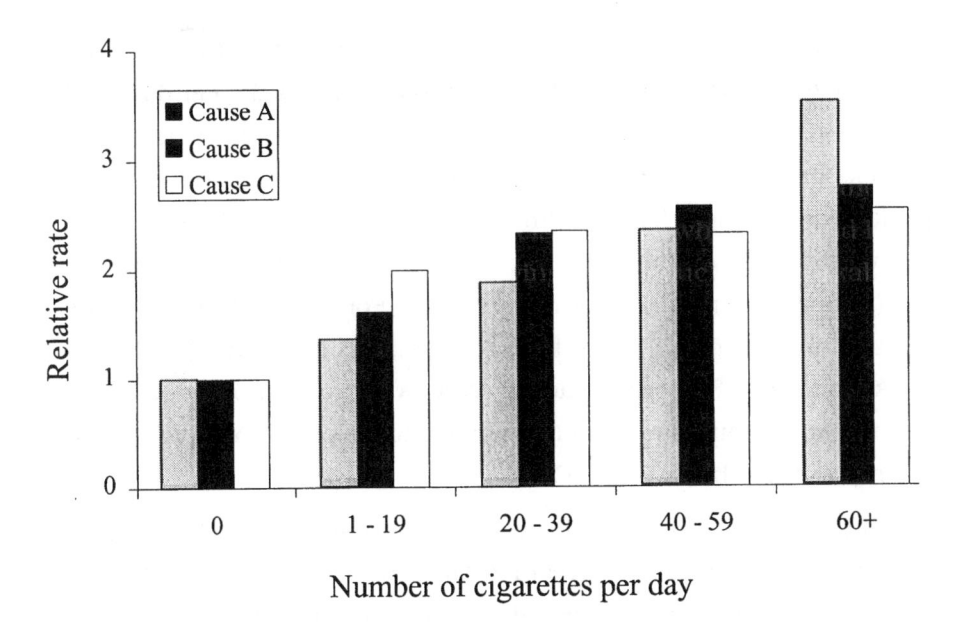

Figure 3

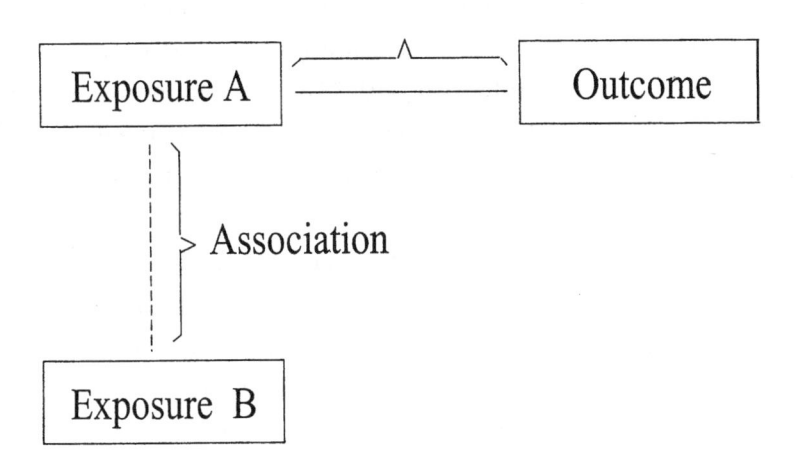

Exposure A (for example, smoking) is associated with the outcome (lung cancer risk); exposure B (yellow fingers) is associated with exposure A - and hence to the outcome

Figure 4

the death rate of the non smokers (i.e. 40% higher rate); the men who smoked 20-39 cigarettes per day (1 to less than 2 packs per day) had 1.9 times the risk; the men who smoked 40-59 cigarettes (2 to less than 3 packs per day) had 2.3 times the risk and the men who smoked 3 packs a day or more had 3.4 times the risk. For cause of death B the equivalent relative rates were 1.5; (less than a pack); 2.3 (1-2 packs); 2.5 (2-3 packs) and 2.7 (3 or more packs). For cause of death C the relative rates were 2.0; (less than a pack); 2.3 (1-2 packs); 2.3 (2-3 packs) and 2.4 (3 or more packs). Now with your knowledge of the health consequences of smoking which causes of death do you think are represented by A, B and C?

C, which shows an increase in risk from non-smokers to less than a pack a day smokers, but little increase after this, is coronary heart disease. B which shows steadily increasing risk with increasing smoking, to a final risk about two and a half times that of non-smokers, is stroke. Cause of death A, which also shows a steadily increasing risk with increasing smoking, but to a final risk about three and a half times that of non-smokers is not (as you may have thought) lung cancer; it is suicide.[5] This is not a chance finding; it has been reported from a series of studies[6], and unlike the p=0.05 effects commonly reported the level of statistical significance is considerably more stringent (p<0.0001). What is likely to be happening here is a mixture of confounding and reverse causation. By confounding we mean that the potential risk factor of interest — smoking — is linked to another factor which in turn is a cause of the outcome. The conventional exposition of confounding refers to the cause of death not included in Figure 3 — lung cancer. This shows a much stronger (and certainly causal) dose-response association with cigarette smoking, with a relative rate of more than 10 among smokers of two packs of cigarettes a day.[7] Smoking causes people to acquire yellow fingers; thus in an observational epidemiological study yellow fingers would be associated with smoking and a naive interpretation would consider yellow fingers as a potential cause of lung cancer (Figure 4).

In the case of our example, if people who are depressed, poor, alcoholic or chronically ill are more likely to be smokers, then as these states increase the risk of suicide, smoking will be non-causally associated with suicide. Taking away the cigarettes from smokers will not, in this case, reduce their risk of suicide (indeed for depressed people who smoke to relieve stress it may increase their risk).

Given the strength of anti-smoking feeling in public health — discussed by Petr frequently, and considered below in the section on epidemiological moralism — it is perhaps not surprising that even though the paper reporting the smoking-suicide association was subtitled "illustration of an artefact from observational epidemiology" it has been widely taken to illustrate that smoking does indeed cause suicide. Biological mechanisms through which this could act — e.g. smoking suppressing brain serotonin levels — have been advanced and a meta-analysis (another *bete noire* of Petr's) has been performed, showing that most studies show the same thing. To address this we looked at an even less plausible cause of death — homicide. Smokers of two packs or more per day were more than twice as likely to be murdered as non-smokers. Unless the provisional wing of the health education lobby has moved on to a direct action phase, during which they shoot smokers, this association is very unlikely to be causal.

The strategy of epidemiologists to deal with confounding is generally statistical "adjustment" or "control", leaving an estimate of the "independent effect" of the risk factor of interest. In theory this sounds an excellent solution, but unfortunately it is of limited use. In the example of smoking and suicide we controlled for a variety of other risk factors (income, ethnicity, chronic disease) all of which are potential confounders and this had almost no effect on the finding (the relative risk for three or more packs a day changed from 3.4 to 3.3 on such adjustment). Not only are there missing variables (e.g. depression) but also the variables which are measured (e.g. income) are measured with error, leaving a wide scope for residual confounding to exist after statistical adjustment.[8]

Black boxes

Petr considered risk factor epidemiology a form of "black box" thinking, as the causal mechanism between exposure and disease is unknown and may even be considered irrelevant (chapter 14). Some epidemiologists consider that epidemiology is most useful when it ventures into territories unconstrained by biological knowledge, since it is here that it may stumble upon novel findings of public health importance.[9] Many epidemiologists, conversely, feel that the future of epidemiology must lie in a rapprochement with biomedical science. Certainly to Petr epidemiology without biology was nonsense; he himself moved from neurotoxicology research (particularly relating to substance P) to his particular blend of "natural scientist, forensic toxicologist, doctor of medicine and connoisseur of the absurd" (as the original footnote to chapter 12 — Smoking and Society read.)

The "black box" nature of risk-factor epidemiology may be particularly evident where low level risks are being investigated. The problems of chance and particularly confounding are exacerbated when the exposure-disease associations are weak. It can be demonstrated that only a small degree of measurement error in a confounder can generate residually confounded effects of the magnitude under consideration for low level radiation, electromagnetic fields around power lines or mobile phones and cancer, for example. As Petr discussed, in many cases these associations may also be biologically implausible, although it must be recognised that what is biologically plausible and what is not changes over time.

An example of the malleable nature of biological plausibility is demonstrated by two epidemiological studies which appeared within a few weeks of each other in 1991. In one study, of Kenyan prostitutes, oral contraceptive use was independently related to risk of future infection with HIV.[10] The authors suggested several mechanisms through which oral contraceptives could facilitate HIV transmission, including a direct effect on the genital mucosa, making it a less successful barrier to HIV, or an immunosuppressive action which increases susceptibility to HIV. Biological knowledge of the effects of oral contraceptives support both these possibilities. The second study, however, found the exact opposite: a protective effect of oral contraceptives on HIV transmission.[11] The authors again found a biologically-supported mechanism for this effect: oral contraceptives thicken the cervical mucus, which then hampers the entry of HIV into the uterine cavity.

As one of his examples of moralism misinterpreted as science Petr quoted a study of cervical cancer which suggested that masturbation was a risk factor (see chapter 7). The author of this study was, however, not hindered from producing an apparent biological mechanism: the pathways from the nervous system to cervical tissue could promote cancer if stimulated.[12]

Clearly apparent "biological plausibility" adds little strength to epidemiological conviction, but equally epidemiology without rapprochement with biology can produce long lists of spurious associations and make no contribution to furthering our understanding of disease aetiology and strategies for disease prevention. An important recent example of how epidemiologists and biologists working together have led to important advances in understanding both epidemiological and biological aspects of disease is seen in the "fetal programming" field.[13] Here initial ecological associations between indices of poor early-life development earlier this century and current disease rates indicated the possible importance of in utero and early childhood growth for later health. These ecological studies were followed by analytical epidemiological studies showing that at an individual level low birthweight and other indices of suboptimal fetal development were related to cardiovascular disease risk profiles in adults. Although there was some existing basic research on fetal development and later health this was limited, and the epidemiological work has enormously stimulated this now vibrant field of biological enquiry.[14] This example — of epidemiology and basic research feeding off each other — illustrates the weaknesses of both "black box" epidemiology and also of those who deny that epidemiology can contribute in a fundamental way to our understanding of disease. Petr's response to the fetal origins work — much of which has occurred since his death — would have greatly interested me, and as in so many areas I miss the opportunity of discussing the issues with him.

Public Health moralism

Petr used to like quoting H L Mencken's comment that hygiene — the public health of its day — "is the corruption of medicine by morality. It is impossible to find a hygienist who does not debase his theory of the healthful with a theory of the virtuous". The targets of epidemiology are, as mentioned, often diet, drinking, smoking, recreational drugs, forms of sexual behaviour, tanning, sloth and obesity — and thus health improvement schemes end up endorsing the message "if it tastes good, don't eat it; if it feels good, don't do it". Petr wrote at length about how the focus of preventive medicine always seemed to be on things people enjoy. Sex and smoking are covered in this book (chapters 7, 12 and 13); but elsewhere[15] other pleasures are discussed. Another moral duty emphasised by public health is the duty to be well. Strictures against smoking, drinking and sloth can also be ways to ensure a more productive workforce, a fitter army and a more fertile population: things with which, historically, most states have been much concerned.[16] The advantage of installing the habit of expecting state interference in private life and private behaviours — through the Trojan horse of beneficence — is also not lost on those who want their leadership accepted. Health as duty can lead to unattainable aims, such as the World Health Organisation definition of health as "Not merely the absence of disease or infirmity" but "A state of complete physical and mental and social well-being". In Petr's words[15] this is "the sort of feeling ordinary people may achieve fleetingly during orgasm, or when high on drugs". Certainly, "Health for all by the year 2000" remains a bad joke for the large majority of the population of the world, now we have reached the new millennium and most people still live in poor and unhealthy places.

Health and longevity are, of course, not the only aims of life. As Petr wrote:

There are fates worse than death. Longevity drags if you have buried your children. Poverty, loneliness, incontinence, dependence, and dementia are some of the final rewards. Not everybody hopes for a long life followed by death from boredom. Plato in *The Republic* recalled the gymnastic teacher Herodicus whose skills enabled him to reach old age in a prolonged death struggle. Hesiod's golden race died swiftly, as though in sleep; they had no old age. Why be afraid of sudden death from coronary heart disease if you cannot regret it the day after?

The function of epidemiology is to study associations and to provide hypotheses for experiments. The epidemiologists should inform; they have no right to tell people what they should do. If they start advising government on "population measures", they declare themselves as agents of social control, they become preventionists for whom the interests of the state override the interest of the individual.[17]

The frequent concordance of morality and what passes at any particular time for the science of public health must surely be more than coincidence. In chapter 12 (Smoking and Society) Petr entertainingly summarises the long history of the war against smoking. When we read of James I pamphleteering against tobacco, through to Hitler's vigorous opposition to smoking, the combination of puritanism and self-interest seem clear. The impossibility of separating ethics or morality from science is, however, highlighted by realising that the 100,000 Reichsmark donation Hitler made to the Institute for the Struggle against the Dangers of Tobacco supported the first methodologically strong epidemiological study showing that smoking causes lung cancer.[18][19] Indeed, the relative risk of lung cancer amongst smokers that can be calculated in the 1943 German study, of 16.6[20], is remarkably similar to the relative risk of 16.3 among male heavy smokers that can be calculated from the classic Doll and Hill case-control study.[21]

The fact that researchers working under an appallingly inhumane dictatorship, during which the most basic elements of human morality and decency were abandoned wholesale, could produce high-calibre science is a demonstration of the impossibility of reading the truth or falsity of claims from the values underlying them. The complexity of this issue is reflected in Petr's discussion of electro-convulsive therapy (Chapter 4), where an apparently barbaric treatment — the adoption of which has surely reflected society's view of the moral status of the mad — is not simply dismissed on these grounds (unlike other treatments, whose basis is simply absurd; see chapters 3 and 15).

As Petr wrote with respect to prevailing views in psychiatry, whether psychotherapy (known as "moral treatment" in the past) or somatic treatment predominates as the ruling paradigm depends less on therapeutic results than on the dominant ideology of the profession (chapter 5). With respect to public health he considered that "the issues of preventive medicine have little to do with science, relative risks, and risk factors. They could be more profitably debated within the framework to which they belong - ethics, politics, and vested interests"[17]. In chapter 10 he expands on this view.

The problematic interpenetration of facts and values has recently been highlighted in the epidemiological world in a debate regarding the need to declare potential conflicts of interest. Kenneth Rothman, a leading epidemiological methodologist, has suggested that forcing the declaration of conflicts of interest is akin to McCarthyism in science, and risks mislabelling everyone as potentially unethical.[22] However, there is also strong evidence that financial interests influence what people say. For example, it has been shown that the expressed viewpoints of experts regarding the beneficial effects (or otherwise) of calcium-channel antagonists is strongly related to the financial relationships the authors had with manufacturers of these drugs.[23]

Rothman's belief that scientists can be objective, and objectivity is not something which is bought or sold, is an opinion I feel Petr would have shared. My own view is that transparency is the best policy in such cases.[24] Both non-disclosure of interests or censorship of viewpoints by suppressing publications by those with such interests prevent readers getting an informed and rounded view of the issues. Transparency in this regard recognises the impossibility of separating facts and values.

Epidemiology as an asocial science

There has been considerable recent debate regarding the focus of much epidemiology on the lifestyles or physiological profiles of people abstracted from their social context.[25][26][27] These authors — in my view correctly — point out that there are broader social determinants of the risks to health that people suffer, and that attempts to reduce these risks should recognise this fundamental social determination. Others have strongly taken issue with this view.[28] Petr recognised the important role of poverty in determining health — referring to the fact that medicine brought many benefits, he considered that the "fact that these achievements have had little or no bearing on the lives of all those millions of our fellows which are still "nasty, poor, brutish, solitary and short" is an indictment of our selfish world"[16]. He was unwilling to allow this admission of the importance of social disadvantage to influence public policy decisions regarding health, however. As he wrote in *The Death of Humane Medicine*:

> Those on the left would argue that trying to change people's lifestyles, without changing the social and commercial pressures which force people to live unhealthy lives, is doomed to failure and results only in victim-blaming. For example, the poor are known to suffer more from diseases and have shorter life expectancy, but should this be blamed on their lifestyle or on the political conditions which are the causes of poverty? Because this kind of analysis appears to be 'well-meaning' in its social concern, it hides its political motive. By linking poverty with disease (which is not unreasonable on its own), Marxists promise that in a classless society the health of the poor will improve. This has not been the experience of the working class in communist countries. Furthermore, the Left, in their various health manifestos, propose increased powers to prescribe healthy activities and proscribe unhealthy activities.

The Right, on the other hand, is more concerned about the 'nation' than about the individual. To maintain the nation in a high state of readiness to defend the supremacy of the race, people should be responsible for their own health. More often, the argument is presented in health-economic terms. To look after the sick is expensive. Patients 'should be made to pay', particularly when most diseases are now said to be 'caused' by unhealthy lifestyles. Typical political statements are contained in Department of Health documents which see health as a matter over which the individual has control and responsibility. It makes little difference to the citizen whether statements such as the list of national targets for physical activity in England, issued by the Faculty of Public Health Medicine in February 1993, emanate from the Left or the Right, as in either case the citizen is threatened by the tyranny of the majority, if he chooses not to fulfil his quota of exercise.

Criticism and the advance of knowledge

Some recent writings about the "limits of epidemiology" have raised ways in which we could do things better than we have in the past. Petr was not interested in playing this game, indeed in a *Lancet* editorial he dismissed a methodological paper I co-authored about improving the design of epidemiological studies[29], which made the modest proposal that more rigorous measurement of exposures on smaller samples contributes more to the production of meaningful findings than more but poorer measures of exposure on larger samples by quoting the Irish country saying "you cannot make a pig grow by weighing him"[30]. In chapter 1, as in *Follies and Fallacies in Medicine* [16], he defended destructive criticism as a necessary cleansing act, which then allowed the building of useful knowledge:

> A critical appraisal of a medical theory takes so much time and effort that most people (and some of them wise) do not bother. It is like an archaeological dig — the slow painstaking search for nuggets of truth by removing layer after layer of deposits left behind by fly-by-night scholars, of dust from the "dry-run" research, of debris left by

those who would rather publish than perish in the rat race, of crumbled clay from the legs of the colossal cacademics carrying the dogma on their shoulders....".

An illustration of the importance of such criticism is provided by the fact that, as I write this preface, the British newspapers are full of reports based on a recent *Lancet* paper[31] suggesting that breast cancer screening with mammography is not a useful preventive strategy. Fifteen years prior to this paper Petr had provided a devastating critique of breast cancer screening (chapter 2), also in the *Lancet* which was, remarkably, not referenced by the more recent paper. It seems that the cleansing act of criticism is required as much today as it was when Petr was writing. He was, in the title of his review of Richard Feynman's memoirs (chapter 16), a subversive man. Epidemiology, public health and medicine generally, still have much to learn from Petr's writings, as the spectre of nonsensus consensus still lingers over us.

Acknowledgements

Many thanks to Liz Humphries for help in preparing this manuscript.

References

1. Poole C, Rothman KJ. Our conscientious objection to the epidemiology wars. J Epidemiol Community Health. 1998;52:613-614.

2. Le Fanu J. The rise and fall of modern medicine. New York: Little Brown, 1999.

3. Mayes LC, Horwitz RI, Feinstein AR. A collection of 56 topics with contradictory results in case-control research.
International Journal of Epidemiology 1989;3:725-7.

4. Oakes M. Statistical Inference. Chichester: Wiley, 1986.

5. Davey Smith G, Phillips AN, Neaton JD. Smoking as "independent" risk factor for suicide: illustration of an artifact from observational epidemiology? *Lancet* 1992;340:709-712.

6. Egger M, Schneider M, Davey Smith G. Spurious precision? Meta-analysis of observational studies. *BMJ* 1998;316:140-4.

7. Davey Smith G, Phillips AN. Passive smoking and health: should we believe Philip Morris's "experts"? *BMJ* 1996;313:929-33.

8. Davey Smith G, Phillips AN. Confounding in epidemiological studies: why "independent" effects may not be all they seem. *BMJ* 1992;305:757-759.

9. Savitz DA. In Defense of Black Box Epidemiology. *Epidemiology* 1994;5:550-552.

10. Plummer FA, Simonsen JN, Cameron DW, Ndinya-Achola JO, Kreiss JK, Gakinya MN, et al. Cofactors in male-female sexual transmission of human immunodeficiency virus type 1.
Journal of Infectious Diseases 1991;163:233-9.

11. Lazzarin A, Saracco A, Musicco M, Nicolosi A. Man-to-woman sexual transmission of the human immunodeficiency virus. *Arch Intern Medicine* 1991;151:2411-6.

12. Rotkin ID. Sexual characteristics of a cervical cancer population. *Am Journal Public Health* 1967;57:815-29.

13. Barker DJP. Mothers, babies and health in later life. London: Churchill Livingstone, 1998.

14. Nathanielsz PW. Life in the womb: the origin of health and disease. New York: Promethean Press, 1999.

15. Skrabanek P. The death of humane medicine. London: The Social Affairs Unit, 1994.

16. Skrabanek P, McCormick J. Follies and Fallacies in Medicine. Third Edition. Whithorn: Tarragon Press 1998.

17. Skrabanek P. Preventive medicine and morality. *Lancet*, 1986:i ;143-144.

18. Schairer E, Schöniger E. Lungenkrebs and Tabakverbrauch. *Zeitschrift fur Krebsforschung* 1943;54:261-9.

19. Davey Smith G, Ströbele SA, Egger M. Smoking and health promotion in Nazi Germany.
Journal of Epidemiology and Community Health 1994;48:220-3.

20. Davey Smith G, Ströbele S, Egger M. Smoking and death.
BMJ 1995;310:396.

21. Doll R, Hill AB. A study of the aetiology of carcinoma of the lung.
BMJ 1952;ii :1271-1287.

22. Rothman JK. Conflict of Interest. The New McCarthyism in Science.
JAMA, 1993:269;2782-2784.

23. Stelfox HT, Chua G, O'Rourke K, Detsky AS. Conflict of interest in the debate over calcium-channel antagonists.
The New England Journal of Medicine, 1998:338;101-106.

24. Smith R. Beyond conflict of interest. Transparency is the key.
BMJ 1998;317:291-2.

25. Diez-Roux AV. Bringing context back into epidemiology: variables and fallacies in multilevel analysis.
American Journal of Public Health, 1998:88;216-222.

26. Koopman JS, Lynch JW. Individual causal models and population system models in epidemiology.
American Journal of Public Health, 1999:89;1170-1174.

27. Krieger N. Epidemiology and the web of causation: has anyone seen the spider? *Social Science and Medicine*, 1994:39;887-903.

28. Rothman KJ, Adami HO, Trichopoulos D. Should the mission of epidemiology include the eradication of poverty? *Lancet*, 1998:352;810-813.

29. Phillips AN, Davey Smith G. The design of prospective epidemiological studies: more subjects or better measurements?
J Clin Epidemiol, 1993;46:1203-1211.

30. Skrabanek P. The epidemiology of errors. *The Lancet*, 1993:342;1502.

31. Gøtzsche PC, Olsen O. Is screening for breast cancer with mammography justifiable? *Lancet*, 2000:355;129-134.

1

IN DEFENCE OF DESTRUCTIVE CRITICISM

(A Dialogue between a Critic C and an Apologist A in an Unnamed Medical School)

C.   I propose that we exchange our usual roles. It is your habit to accuse me of destructive criticism. On this occasion let me defend criticism against your attack, destructive as it may be.

A: You know that I hate to be destructively critical; it is your perverse pleasure. Lucifer is the patron saint of your negativistic revolt. Ortega y Gasset was right when he said that the only true revolt is creation — the revolt against nothingness [1].

C.   Don't quote Ortega y Gasset as the Devil quotes the Bible. Ortega spoke as a philosopher; he was not concerned with the refutation of medical theories.

A: I grant you that he did not speak as a scientist. His point, nevertheless, does not lose its sharpness. To create ideas is a positive activity, while you, on the other hand, seem to enjoy demolishing what others have built with love.

C: You know the story about Potemkin, the lover of Catherine II. She entrusted him with money with which to improve the muzhiks' lot. Potemkin squandered the money on pleasure instead of using it for building villages as he was expected to do. When Catherine went to inspect them, Potemkin fooled her by hastily having erected only the front walls facing the road along which her equipage was to travel. I suspect that you prefer instinctively Potemkin's villages to an empty space. Why not pull the sham gables down? How could you criticise Potemkin's constructions constructively?

This paper first appeared in *Perspectives in Biology and Medicine*, 30, 1 Autumn 1986
© 1986 by the University of Chicago. All rights reserved.
Reproduced by kind permission of The University of Chicago Press

A: You are not being fair. Your Potemkin's village is a case of the Emperor's New Clothes. There is nothing wrong with calling a sham a sham. What I mean is something different. God created a beautiful world, and it was Lucifer who was jealous.

C. What on earth was there for Lucifer to create? An anti-Creation? He only refused to sing praises. Besides, scientific theories and God's creation have little in common, metaphors aside. Even the highest achievements of the human mind have no eternal validity. Look what happened to Newton's laws, believed by Kant to be a priori true. Einstein put an end to it.

A: Einstein was not out to get Newton, mind you. It was not a question of sour grapes. He *improved* on Newton. That's what constructive criticism is about.

C: It's all very well, if you are an Einstein — the best armchair researcher, by the way, we've ever had. But what about the lesser mortals, like ourselves. Listen to this short passage from John Locke, who makes the point ever so humbly: "The commonwealth of learning is not at this time without master-builders, whose mighty designs, in advancing the sciences, will leave lasting monuments to the admiration of posterity; but everyone must not hope to be a Boyle or a Sydenham; and in the age that produces such masters as the great Huygenius and the incomparable Mr. Newton, with some others of that strain, it is ambition enough to be employed as an under-labourer in clearing the ground a little, and removing some of the rubbish that lies in the way of knowledge" [2].

A: You are groping for straws. You try to justify your malicious joy in destroying the work of others.

C: Not a good work, which I admire as much as you do. However, one should be permitted to identify error without being required to correct it. Everyone would profit from it. The weeding out and extermination of pests are not pleasurable activities, but they serve to enhance the pleasures of a well-kept garden. Why shouldn't one be free to say that a piano is out of tune, without knowing how to tune it, or, to take it a step further, to tune a piano without being able to play it;

or take faultfinding — is that a "negative" activity?

A: I accept that it has its place. Checking a plane for faults before a takeoff may be as important for a safe flight as the ability of the pilot to fly it. But you don't care whether the plane crashes. You are bent on debunking.

C: Debunking is a funny word. Do you know it was first used after a member for Buncombe County used to make long speeches in the Congress to impress his constituency? Deflating windbags is a cheap sport that does not interest me.

A: Debunking or destructive criticism, call it what you will. You cannot deny that it is easier than creative thought.

C: Bunkum! A critical appraisal of a medical theory takes so much time and effort that most people (and some of them wise) do not bother. It is like an archaeological dig — the slow painstaking search for nuggets of truth by removing layer after layer of deposits left behind by fly-by-night scholars, of dust from the "dry-run" research, of debris left by those who would rather publish than perish in the rat race, of crumbled clay from the legs of the colossal cacademics carrying the dogma on their shoulders....

A: You are cynical as always.

C: The Cynics were watchdogs terrifying malefactors. They tried to expose falseness and conceit. That's why their name is still spoken with a snarl. But let me finish. You excavate the droppings of parrots and the petrified turds, and, when the dust settles, where is a Troy to feast your eye on? Do you call this a pleasure? How much easier is a creative thought, such as that food is the cause of heart disease, breast cancer, or piles? It comes in a flash of inspiration. There are thinkers who father such ideas as that, barring accidents, smoking and sex explain all remaining diseases that cannot be accounted for by dietary indiscretions and by drinking. Simplicity has an irresistible appeal.

A: You are trivialising everything. Take, for example, smoking. The U.S. Surgeon-General has 40,000 references, results of millions of man-hours of research, to prove that smoking is one of the most serious health hazards known.

C.   Has it ever struck you that, if the Surgeon-General was right, he would not need to boast with an army of 40,000 papers? This is the whirl of dust I spoke of. A useful smoke screen to obscure the facts.

A: You can't be serious. How can you doubt the most ironclad truth of epidemiological research. Every child knows it's true.

C: Georg Lichtenberg said 200 years ago that the most ardent advocates of a doctrine are those who are not fully familiar with the facts and who are secretly aware of their deficiency [3]. But I'd like to return to what you call "destructive" criticism. There is a passage from Trotter I'd like to read you first: "The common tendency to regard destructive criticism as always easy and generally reprehensible is one that I do not share; indeed, I doubt if it could be acquiesced in by any sensible person making a frank survey of the intellectual world today. We cannot but be struck by the remarkable prevalence of systems of doctrine, by their loudness, their confusion, and their deleterious effect on conduct. In all these systems the most indulgent examination will find little evidence of really enterprising thought, but it will find a great deal of reconditioned lumber, at its best of a low order of reality and now used to justify the lazier, the uglier, and the baser inclinations of the human spirit. At no time in the history of the intellect has the sanitary work of destructive criticism been more needful" [4].

A: I think that you're unduly selective in your quotations. In medicine, anyway, destructive criticism is irresponsible, for it may deprive patients of proper treatment.

G: Or save their lives, if the treatment is improper. *Primum non nocere* does not mean do no harm to doctors' dogmas, but do not harm the patients. Unfortunately, if you criticise a medical theory, the author takes it personally, rather than disown his aborted thought.

A: You revel in acting devil's advocate, finding a pleasure in being unpleasant. *Le plaisir aristocratique de déplaire*, eh?

C: Let me remind you that *advocatus diaboli* was a jocular term for the office of *promotor fidei*. Nothing devilish in pointing out flaws in the evidence adduced by the postulators. He was not against canonisation of a candidate for sainthood; he acted only as a quality-control man so that a fatal mistake would not have been committed by canonising an unworthy person. Similarly in medicine: the more harm you can cause by your theory, the better the devil's advocate you should hire. If in doubt, admit ignorance, tell the truth. This is known, unfortunately, as fouling your own nest.

A: I don't like your scatological metaphor. You seem to have been reading too much Chargaff lately.

C: You pronounce his name as if it were Satan's. His work on nucleic acids was monumental; he was creative. wasn't he? This did not stop him from saying that "reason and judgement should not abdicate when faced with a dogma. It is imperative that the most stringent criticism be applied to tentative scientific hypotheses that disguise themselves as dogmas. This criticism must come from within; but it can only come from an outsider at the inside" [5]. To be sure, he was talking about science and not medicine. About cancer research he said that, because it spreads like cancer, it has become the best model of cancer itself.

A: Such sweeping statements serve no purpose. We are getting cancer under control.

C: I am keeping my mind open, but not to the extent that my brains fall out.

A: You are a liquidator of ideas.

C: Yes, if you use the word in its original sense, I mean, someone who wants to clarify, to make transparent.

A: You are just playing with words. What I mean is that you are a negativist, that you do not strive for positive truths.

C: You are also playing with words. Truth is neither negative nor positive. To show that a person has not got a disease with which he is falsely labelled does not amount to a "negative" truth; it makes the "patient" positively healthy. To expose a liar is a positive act: it is the liar who spreads "negative" truths, that is, lies.

In Defence of Destructive Criticism

A: Enough of your verbal tricks. What I am talking about is negative criticism for its own sake.

C: I am not sure what you mean by "negative" criticism, which I presume you use as a synonym for "destructive" criticism. It sounds to me like a pleonasm, a tautology, like a dialogue between two persons. Effective criticism, in negating a false idea, is always destructive of that idea. If it were refutable it would not be destructive. Irrefutable criticism brings bad news.

A: Why not offer a friendly criticism?

C: Such as, I find your ideas extremely interesting and fascinating except that your basic premises are wrong? I hope that you do not mean by friendly criticism the type, "Oh, you wicked, wicked little thing," which Alice applied to her kitten, while kissing it in order to make the kitten understand that it was in disgrace. The spectre of destructive criticism is always raised by the defender of dogma at the very moment when he runs out of arguments.

A: You know very well that by destructive criticism I mean criticism without offering an alternative, constructive solution.

C: This is a useful dodge with which to escape any criticism.

A: What do you mean?

C: Well, let's suppose that a psychiatrist comes to you with a theory that the moon, or a neuropeptide, is causing mental disease. Why should not a rational criticism of such a thesis be perfectly acceptable, even though you, or anyone else, may have no clue as to what is the cause of mental disease. If a man is drowning in his own nonsense, you should pull him out first, before you start teaching him how to swim. Even if you do not know how to swim, or how to teach swimming, you still have to pull him out.

A: You are an iconoclast, aren't you?

C: The pejorative flavour of this term is due to the fact that the opponents of iconoclasts — let's call them iconoblasts — won their right to venerate holy pictures in the ninth century and have been in power since. But don't forget that the iconoclasts were equally dogmatic. Iconoclasm has no place in science because science has nothing to venerate. But in religion or medicine, that's a different matter.

A: I find your allusions to religion curious.

C: You use them as often as I do. Unfortunately, the religious metaphor pervades our evaluation of medical theories. We speak of dogma, orthodoxy, and heretical views as if those who cling to the current dogma were morally better than nonbelievers. Nietzsche once suggested that it is not their love for men but the impotence of their love that hinders the Christians of today from burning those who do not agree with them [6].

A: I am not surprised that you admire Nietzsche, but it is an exaggeration that medical authorities wish to persecute their critics.

C: Thomas Szasz, whose writing is a paragon of clear thought and whose ideas have stirred psychiatry from its dogmatic slumbers, was accused of not "believing" in mental illness, and the Commissioner of the New York State Department of Mental Hygiene demanded that he be dismissed from his university position as a professor of psychiatry [7].

A: One swallow does not make a summer. In the end you have to take sides and believe something. You cannot equivocate all the time.

C: In this you are mistaken. Ignorance is preferable to dogma. We do not have to believe, but we often do. For some it is less painful and more consoling than to remain suspended in midair on a string of doubts. There is only one dogma in science: do not blindly believe in any dogma.

A: But this is your belief! Your dogma is the value of criticism that is destructive. Therefore you also believe something.

C: Your argument reminds me of the fundamentalists who argue that if creationism is prohibited from being taught in the schools, so should be the "religion" of secular humanism.

A: I am not talking about religious beliefs. However, I can't see how you can escape from the fact that even you have to have some dogmatic beliefs.

C: Perhaps our misunderstanding stems from the two different senses of "belief": acceptance of something as true without sufficient evidence and a readiness to act on the basis of information that may be false.

A: The distinction sounds somewhat specious to me. Can you give me an example?

C: Well. if I were to travel by train tonight from Dublin to Cork, I would go to the station at the appointed time, because I would "believe" that the train would be there. If, on the other hand, you asked me, Do you believe in the truth that the train will leave the station tonight at a given time? I would most certainly say no.

A: But if you had travelled by the same train every night for 20 years, would you not come to believe that the train always leaves at the same time?

G: Not necessarily. I think it was Wittgenstein who pointed out that, by buying another copy of the same newspaper, you will not verify the truthfulness of a statement printed in it.

A: This is another of your silly witticisms, irrelevant to what I am saying. Independent confirmations of a theory strengthen its validity.

C: Or permit the same sin with an increasing sense of pending absolution. Weak independent confirmations will certainly help to create consensus, which is, as a rule, a unison of the loudest voices drowning the discordant squeaks. Truth is not decided by a majority vote. When bloodletting was a panacea, its curative value was confirmed repeatedly and independently and vouched for by centuries of experience. Even patients were convinced.

A: What has this anachronistic example to do with what we are talking about?

C: If you want a contemporary example, take the latest consensus on the diet-heart question agreed on by the National Institutes of

Health, or, if that is too fanciful, cervical cancer screening.

A: There is no controversy about that.

C: That is true, despite the fact that we have not a single study that actually tests the assumption that screening saves lives. I admit that it would not be an easy undertaking in the present climate, when they ram the belief down your throat without letting you even gag. I have made a list of unanswered questions about cervical screening and sent it off to a well-known medical journal. The editor got cold feet: "not balanced," you know; it was not "constructive" criticism. For each pinprick of criticism you are supposed to provide a salve that will heal it. ABC said XYZ, while CBA said ZYX—this is known in the trade as a nice balanced review. The editors go mad for it. But I was not doing any balancing act, I was just asking questions; and I still wait for answers.

A: Why are you always on the lookout for negative instances and counterarguments?

C: Because it is the quickest way to learn. As Popper says, valid criticism consists in pointing out that a theory does not provide the goodies it has promised to deliver. I do not look for contradictions for their own sake — as you are imputing to me all the time — but because they demarcate more sharply the boundaries of our ignorance. The faster you go through the mistakes, the quicker you move toward more solid knowledge [8].

A: I am surprised that you are prepared to believe in the growth of knowledge at all.

C: The path is unlighted and rough but safer than the treacherous boglands of dogma that surround it. What you call "destructive criticism" is only the outstretched hand of a weary traveller trying to save a fellow man from disappearing in the quagmire of unfounded certainty.

A: And what is the destination of your traveller, may I ask?

C: He will die on the road.

References

1. Ortega y Gasset J. Mission of the University. Kegan Paul, London, 1946.

2. Locke J. An Essay Concerning Human Understanding. London: Oxford Univ. Press. 1894 (Originally published 1690).

3. Lichtenberg GC. Gedanken, Satiren. Fragmente, vol. 1, edited by W. Herzog. Diederich, Jena, 1907.

4. The Collected Papers of Wilfred Trotter, F.R.S. Oxford Univ. Press, London, 1941.

5. Chargaff, E. Essays on Nucleic Acids. Elsevier, Amsterdam, 1963.

6. Nietzsche, F. Jenseits von Gut und Böse [(Beyond good and evil), translated by R. J. Hollingdale. Penguin, London, 1973. (originally published 1886.)]

7. Szasz, T. The Myth of Mental Illness. Paladin, London, 1972.

8. Popper, K. R. Objective Knowledge: An Evolutionary Approach. Oxford University Press, London, 1972.

2

FALSE PREMISES AND FALSE PROMISES OF BREAST CANCER SCREENING

The evidence that breast cancer is incurable is overwhelming. The philosophy of breast cancer screening is based on wishful thinking that early cancer is curable cancer, though no-one knows what is "early". Unable to admit ignorance and defeat, cancer propagandists have now turned to blaming the victims: they consume too much fat, they do not practise breast self-examination, they succumb to "irrational" fears and delay reporting the early symptoms. It would appear that no woman needs to die of breast cancer if she reads and heeds the leaflets of the cancer societies and has her breasts examined regularly. Adherence to these myths and avoidance of reality undermines the credibility of the medical profession with the public.

Natural history and curability of breast cancer

Breast cancer is the commonest cancer in women: by the age of 75, between 6% and 10% have clinical breast cancer.[1] It is about ten times more common than cervical cancer; and, if screening for cancer could reduce the case-fatality rate, breast cancer should be top of the list for screening.

Natural History

Since surgical treatment for breast cancer has been available for more than 100 years, there is scant information on unoperated cases. Bloom et al[2] reviewed 250 cases of untreated breast cancer from the period between 1805 and 1933. Only 35% of these cancers were histologically documented, but the great majority were in stage III or IV (97.5%). Surprisingly, after 5 years 20% were still alive, and 5% survived 10

This paper first appeared with the title 'Screening for Disease: False Premises and False Promises of Breast Cancer Screening', in *The Lancet* 1985; ii: 316-320. © The Lancet Ltd. Reproduced by kind permission of The Lancet Ltd.

years. The cumulative survival curve in Bloom's series exhibited a peculiar pattern of decreasing mortality with time. This paradoxical decrease in the force of mortality with time has also been observed in treated cancers.[3,4] Another oddity in the natural history of breast cancer is that very large tumours (>6 cm) have better survival rates than smaller tumours.[3] Breast cancer is not a nosological entity: Gallager[5] listed more than twenty pathological categories. Some of the variants metastasise rarely and have an excellent prognosis — eg, tubular ductal carcinoma, which represents about 10% of the tumours.[6]

Another piece of evidence regarding the natural history of breast cancer is analysis of tumour doubling times. Most tumours are detected when their diameter is more than 1 cm (which is about the limit of palpability), but even at this "early" stage the tumour contains 5×10^8 cells, requiring 29 binary divisions from the initial single cancer cell. At the fastest doubling time recorded in one series (109 days) — on the assumption that growth was linear — it would take 8-9 years to reach this stage,[7] at which, however, many breast cancers have already metastasised.[8] Bauer et al[9] estimated that 90% of tumours have metastasised by the time the tumour reaches a volume of 125 µl and a diameter of 6 mm. For breast cancer discovered between annual screenings ("interval cancers") the doubling time is 30-70 days.[10] "As many as 77% of all breast cancers may grow fast enough to grow from below the threshold size detectable on mammograms to clinically detectable size in less than 12 months."[11] The long survival of some patients, whether treated or untreated, suggests a slow growth of some tumours. The slowest doubling time recorded by Buchanan et al[7] was 944 days. Von Fournier et al[12] observed breast cancers with the tumour volume doubling time as long as 5 years and as short as 44 days. Unexpectedly, there was no correlation between the doubling time and the histological grade.

Claims of "cure" in studies with a short follow-up time — ie, less than 30-40 years—are unjustified.[13-17]

Finally, evidence on the natural history is supplemented by necropsy findings. As many as 6% of women dying of other causes have breast carcinoma in situ and 20% have dysplasia.[18] In 83 consecutive necropsies in women older than 20 years, Nielsen et al[19] found that 21 (25%) had invasive breast carcinoma or premalignant lesions. These figures hide a large potential for overdiagnosis and overtreatment.

Curability of Breast Cancer

If breast cancer is incurable, as many surgeons believe, then screening only adds years of anxiety and fear. The current controversy between the advocates of maximal and minimal surgery — ie, between the "radicals" and the "conservatives" — stems from their respective beliefs as to the local or systemic nature of breast cancer. This is not a new division.

In 1888, Jackson commented upon the lack of evidence that simple mastectomy is inferior to more radical operations, which, at his time, included removal of all axillary nodes (Banks), clearance of the whole axilla (Gross), removal of supraclavicular lymph nodes (Owens), or removal of the upper limb at the shoulder joint (Esmarch), in addition to total mastectomy. Jackson thought that these more radical operations were "unscientific and needlessly cruel to many women" and he warned against ignoring clinical experience which had shown that radical surgery did not defer recurrence: "I hope we shall not, ignoring the opinion of (Sir James) Paget as to the constitutional nature of the disease ... wander on the strength of a delusion as to the local nature of the disease."[20] More recently, Baum and Edwards[21] reiterated that introduction of Halsted's operation in 1898 did not make any impact on survival of breast cancer patients. One hundred years on, the same controversy is around, occasionally degenerating into "vituperation, contumely, and vilification"[22] with "claims, counterclaims, and quackery ... admixed heterogeneously in a chaos of doubt".[23] "Enthusiasts put forward widely conflicting views often more notable for dogmatic assertion and vehemence than for logical thought ... These entrenched though widely ranging doctrines have resulted in a most unhappy and confused clinical situation. Many inadequately controlled series have been published, comparing like with unlike and drawing unjustifiable conclusions."[24]

In the published work wishful thinking abounds. For example, Lewison introduced a volume on breast cancer by stating that "we must now be born-again believers and anticipate the golden age of cancer surgery, complemented by radiotherapy, hormone therapy, chemotherapy, and immunotherapy".[25] If we cannot conquer cancer, at least let us give it the full works.

Chemotherapy and endocrine therapy have only a limited and palliative value.[26,27] Fashions in chemotherapy change too fast for allowing a reasonable time to assess them, but rapid changes are themselves indicative of unfulfilled promise. "One must be astonished at the sudden plethora of therapeutic talent, though not without fear of the coming day of reckoning."[28] The common fallacy of comparing "respondents" with "non-respondents" in chemotherapeutical trials was exposed by Oye and Shapiro.[29]

Local mastectomy (with irradiation) was found preferable to radical mastectomy as early as 1928.[30] Although this was recently confirmed,[31,32] we still do not know whether patients survive equally long if the breast is not removed but only irradiated.[33] The value of radiotherapy in early breast cancer remains uncertain.[34] Park and Lees concluded that surgery improved the 5-year survival at best by only 5-10%.[35] Survival rates are little affected by any of the current methods used, whether it be radical or simple mastectomy, with or without radiation, and with or without chemotherapy.[14,22,31,32] Prophylactic resection or irradiation of regional lymph nodes, with or without metastases, does not improve survival.[31,32,36] "It is surely complacent to continue our current practice of subjecting at least 70% of women with primary disease to a futile mutilating procedure."[13] "One thing is certain: survival is much more closely related to the intrinsic malignancy of the tumour than to early diagnosis and treatment."[37]

Aggressiveness is often a sign of desperation, and surgical aggression is no exception. In the USA, in 1977, 50% of breast cancer surgery was the radical (Halsted) procedure, and in 1981, 77% of operations were modified radical mastectomy.[38] Those on the receiving end are not amused: "We can only regard these (surgeons) as the dinosaurs of their profession who are even now, like those ancient monsters, shambling on their way to extinction because their brains are too small to cope with new knowledge."[39] Harsh words, but if our irrational sorties against breast cancer continue, we shall hear more of these unpleasantries.

"Early" intervention as the only hope for cure means little in practice. If "early" means visible, palpable, or symptomatic, then, clearly, it is too late. 20% of "occult" cancers, detectable only by mammography, had metastasised to the axilla.[40] The unrecognised, microscopic metastases from tumours below 1 cm in diameter will on average become clinically demonstrable 10 years later.[3] McKinnon[41] showed that "early" treatment had failed to reduce cancer mortality, but he observed that "early" cases included many lesions of low or no lethal potential. On the other hand, if "early" means premalignant lesions, then it could be too early; evidence must be provided that such lesions would develop into an invasive cancer within the life-span of the bearer, if a potentially large number of unnecessary mastectomies is to be prevented. It is unacceptable to remove breasts on the basis of theoretical speculation.

The earliest possible intervention is removal of a healthy breast. The belief that the fewer organs we have the less likely we are to die is reductio ad absurdum. Contralateral "prophylactic" mastectomy was advocated as early as 1921 by Bloodgood, who used to work with Halsted. The practice still flourishes.[42-44] The zeal of some surgeons for contralateral prophylactic mastectomies betrays their disbelief that "early" cancer is curable — otherwise they would wait till a lesion becomes detectable by mammography. It is known that the development of cancer in the second breast does not influence the overall outcome.[45,46] The actual incidence of contralateral cancer is about 0.5% a year, with about 1-2% discovered simultaneously.[14,15,46] Since the incidence of "histological cancer" in the second breast in random biopsies is 15-25%,[42] many of such lesions cannot have an invasive potential. In the case of intraductal carcinoma in situ (CIS), there is no justification for contralateral mastectomy, since progression, occurring in about 40%, is invariably in the same breast.[47] The malignant potential of lobular CIS is so low that some pathologists prefer the terms "benign neoplasia" or "dysplasia"; it is bilateral in about half the cases; and, though it does not metastasise itself, it predisposes to the subsequent development of invasive carcinoma, which occurs as often in the contralateral breast as in the one in which the CIS was originally diagnosed.[10] There is no evidence that early mastectomy affects survival. If the patients knew this, they would most likely refuse surgery.[41]

The logic of breast cancer treatment, or rather the lack of it, can be illustrated by an imaginary dialogue (inspired by Kardinal and Yarbro[50]) between a dogmatist (D), shielded by "conceptual rationalisation" (brilliantly exposed by Baum[49]) and an empiricist (E) who judges the theory by its fruits:

D: Early detection is surest protection.
E: From what?
D: From dying of disseminated cancer.
E: We know that breast cancer disseminates long before it is clinically detectable.
D: Early cancer is a localised disease.
E: Why then do even your stage-I patients succumb if they are followed for long enough?
D: They either get a new breast cancer or they were wrongly staged. I never take chances and, like Halsted, I cut it all out.
E: But Americans have just shown that radical mastectomy is no better than simple mastectomy.
D: If you read the reports carefully you will know that with simple mastectomy they irradiated the axilla or used chemotherapy.
E: Existing evidence shows no benefit from radiotherapy or chemotherapy on mortality rates.

D: My dear friend, you are a therapeutic nihilist. To cure cancer, surely, all cancer cells must be removed — first by radical surgery, and then by chemotherapy and radiation to gobble up the occasional cell which has gone astray.

E: But it does not cure the patients.

D: I have always maintained that early detection is the only sure protection.

E: Against what?

(*Exit* Dogmatist, slamming door.)

Screening under scrutiny

There are two screening procedures available: (a) mammography, and (b) breast palpation, either by the doctor or by the woman herself. Of the remaining options, magnetic resonance imaging provides excellent pictures at a prohibitive cost, thermography is unreliable, and ultrasound is insensitive.[51]

Mammography is very expensive: $195,000 per cancer detected[10] or £80 000 for one life saved.[12] Mammography should be supplemented by physical examination if large numbers of false negatives are to be avoided.[53] Breast self-examination (BSE) is the cheapest and the least reliable method.

Specificity and Sensitivity

False-positive results are all those cases in which a suspicious lesion is not confirmed by biopsy as malignant. This is true in about 80-90% of biopsies. An unknown, but probably high, percentage of women who underwent mastectomy for CIS should also be added to the false-positive results, since many such lesions would never have developed into an invasive carcinoma if left alone. False-positives due to misdiagnosis are very common: of 506 small tumours or CIS in the Breast Cancer Detection Demonstration Project (BCDDP), 88 were shown on review to be benign or "borderline".[54] Discrepancy between the rate of mastectomies and breast cancer in the UK also indicates overdiagnosis.[55]

Equally serious is false reassurance due to false-negative results. In the Health Insurance Plan (HIP) study, 40% of breast cancers were missed on mammography.[56] The average false-negative rate for mammography is 10-30%,[7] but could be as high as 73%.[57] Haagensen and Asch[58] noted in their series that the mean delay in 54 patients due to false-negative mammograms was 43 weeks. The sensitivity of BSE is very low: the average size of tumours is 3-4 cm in diameter. In women with health-professional training, the mean tumour size found by BSE was somewhat larger (3.8 cm) than in other women (3.5 cm), indicating that the low sensitivity of BSE is not due to low education.[59]

Screening Intervals

There should be valid information regarding the optimum frequency for screening. In the BCDDP patients, 20-26% of cancers surfaced between annual screenings ("interval cancers").[60,61] In the HIP study, 33% of cancers were interval cancers, and in one study, 77%.[11] Haagensen[10] suggested that, for detecting early stages of all breast cancers, screening would have to be done every 4 months. The interval cancers are more aggressive and their prognosis is worse than that of the cancers detected by screening.

It is agreed that mammography is the only practical test that can detect breast cancer before it is palpable.[63] Early detection does not guarantee cure, though it leads to longer morbidity and longer survival times due to the lead-time bias. This is often confused with better prognosis and lower mortality. Garwin[64] calculated that the "improvement" in 5-year survival rates since 1950, amounting to about 10% for 97% of cancers, can be explained by the fact that cancers are diagnosed an average of 6 months earlier.

Breast Self-examination

Since even mammography does not prevent women dying from breast cancer (at least not in women below age 50), it is dishonest for cancer societies to promulgate BSE as a method for "early" detection. Unfortunately, "to cast any doubt on the goodness and worthiness of BSE somewhat appears sacrilegious, taking a dour scientist's view of this tender, humane, consumer-generated, self-help activity. But this is precisely the scepticism that many physicians had sadly learned from transient fads in the breast-cancer field".[65]

Turner et al[66] found that the mean size of breast cancer tumours was 3.0 cm in the BSE group and 3.2 in the control group. In a population-based prospective study of a cohort of 22,500 women, age-group 45-65, BSE had no effect on the incidence and the stage of presentation of breast cancer.[67] The mean size of all tumours was 3.4 cm (BSE and controls) compared with 3.5 cm in the controls. Both the BSE group and the controls delayed considerably before reporting an abnormality: 52% and 50%, respectively, delayed for more than a month. Frankl and Ackerman[40] noted that "for whatever reasons, the mortality is much higher among those women whose cancers were found by self-examination".

The lack of influence of educational campaigns on the interval between discovery of a lump and consultation had already been noted in 1928 in Philadelphia.[68] The reasons for delay are easy to understand. The delay is a form of denial. The fear of "discovery" may explain why only 30% of invited women in the Huddersfield trial accepted.[67] It is a paradox that the acceptors of BSE should be "rewarded" for their health-conscious self-care by mutilation, still at a stage when they feel healthy. Those who delay reporting are likely to be blamed for their doom, despite the fact that survival is not related to duration of symptoms.[69]

Mammography — Safety and Effectiveness

The requirement that a test be safe is naturally more stringent when a symptom-free population is screened. Informed consent should be the rule but it is rarely sought.

Screening programmes are often publicity exercises with no intention to provide interpretable data. For example, in the BCDDP, which was rushed through in the favourable climate created by the news that the wives of the US President and of the Vice-President had breast cancer, the organisers openly admitted that "the programme was not originally designed as a research or investigational project; no provision was made for systematic collection of data."[61] Over 280,000 women were recruited without being told that no benefit of mammography had been shown in a controlled trial for women below 50, and without being warned about the potential risk of induction of breast cancer by the test which was supposed to detect it.[70] Despite the warning by the committee of the National Academy of Sciences of the USA on the risks, the women were exposed to doses that could cause more cancers in the long run than could be prevented by the programme.[71-73] A glimpse behind the scenes was provided by Greenberg,[74] who quoted a director of the National Cancer Institute as saying: "both the American Cancer Society and the National Cancer Institute will gain a great deal of favourable publicity because they are bringing research findings to the public ... This will assist in obtaining more research funds". A windfall of this shameful affair was a considerable reduction of the risk of cancer induction by mammography, though the risk is still not negligible, particularly in women below 50 in whom mammography gives no benefit.[75-78]

In the latest evaluation of the HIP study, Strax[56] admitted that mammography did not pick up lesions earlier than clinical examination: "79% of the cancers found on the X-ray alone were free of nodal involvement — this compares with 75% on clinical examination alone." At 10-year follow-up, there had been 91 deaths from breast cancer in the mammography group and 128 in the control group. A peculiar finding, not commented upon by the authors, was that the subgroup of women in the mammography group who refused screening (35%) had a lower incidence and mortality due to breast cancer than either the mammography group or the control group.[79] In the initial report it was claimed that 42 carcinomas were detected by mammography only.[62] However, a special committee later found that of "44 carcinomas in the study group reported as having been detected by mammography, 28 were believed to have been present as a dominant mass that was missed in the original examination. In 19 (68%) of the 28, the carcinoma was identified clinically when these patients were re-examined. In 3 other patients in whom mammography detected microcalcification, repeated clinical examination also revealed a palpable tumour."[10] Thus, in the HIP study, mammography detected only 17% of 132 carcinomas in 20,166 women.[10] Despite the huge cost and effort, the HIP project detected only 3% of breast cancers that would be expected to cause death in the lifetime of the study cohort.[80] The maximum benefit of the HIP study (without taking into account the lead-time bias and cancer induction) was 1% fewer breast cancer deaths a year.[10]

The last completed randomised trial from two Swedish counties was 2.5 times larger than the HIP trial, but again it showed no benefit from mammography to the women under the age of 50.[81] Even in the age group 50-74, the benefit was significant only in one of the two counties: only 7 deaths per 10^5 per year were prevented by screening, which amounts to about 0.2% of total deaths expected to occur annually in this age-group. No data have been published so far on interval cancers and on the overall mortality in the study and control groups.

Two recent case-control studies on the value of mammography,[82,83] are hard to interpret because of inherent biases in the methodology.[64] In one of these studies[82] no benefit was shown for women aged 50-54, which contradicts the findings of the randomised trials. It is for these reasons that results of yet another, the Edinburgh randomised trial, which started in 1979 and will take 7 years to complete, are awaited with keen interest.[85]

Public education

Screening programmes, with the accompanying propaganda from cancer societies and media, may heighten the level of cancerophobia in society, with little to show in return. This could have an adverse effect on the credibility of the medical profession. Extensive programmes of cancer detection have no impact on the "earliness" of breast tumours.[86] "Mass media channels alone could only increase anxiety, which achieves nothing unless the means to resolve it are also provided."[87] The psychiatric problems generated by BSE are underrated. Maguire found in his psychiatric practice that there was an increasing number of women who developed an obsessional ritual of self-examination. Patients in whom breast cancer was diagnosed at a stage when it was not palpable lived in fear that they would be unable to tell if there was recurrence. In general, women who have breast cancer discovered by screening while they are still symptom-free, adapt less well to their serious illness.[88]

Many women whose expectations have been pitched by cancer propaganda feel that they are not getting the best medical attention: "They demand us to manage this ourselves ... many times I have thought that if this were something concerning men they would accordingly take measures and tackle it at once. But we are just sitting here feeling our breasts! And yet, if we find a lump, it does not mean that we escape radical mastectomy ... but so then, why are we not demanding mammography?"[89]

The profession has become a prey to its own wishful thinking. In a recent survey of beliefs of general practitioners in Edinburgh and Oxford, about two thirds believed that there is convincing evidence for benefits of BSE, and a further half believed that there is no need for further randomised trials before decisions are made about screening facilities. We should climb off the cancer bandwagon and admit our ignorance.

References

1. Pike MC, Ross RK. Breast Cancer. *Br Med Bull* 1984; 40: 351-54.
2. Bloom HJG, Richardson WW, Hurin EJ. Natural history of untreated breast cancer (1805-1933). Comparison of untreated and treated cases according to histological grade of malignancy. *Br Med J* 1962; ii: 213-21.
3. Duncan W, Kerr GR. The curability of breast cancer. *Br Med J* 1976; ii: 781-83.
4. Zajicek G. On the improving chances of the cancer patient. *Med Hypotheses* 1983; 12: 369-76.

5. Gallager HS. Problems in the classification of breast cancer. *Radiol Clin N Am* 1983; 21:13-26.
6. Carstens PHR. Tubular carcinoma of the breast. A study of frequency. *Am J Clin Pathol* 1978; 70: 204-10.
7. Buchanan JB, Sputt JS, Heuser LS. Tumor growth, doubling times and inability of the radiologist to diagnose certain cancers. *Radiol Clin N Am* 1983; 21: 115-26.
8. Heuser L, Spratt JS, Polk HC, Buchanan J. Relation between mammary cancer growth kinetics and the interval between screenings. *Cancer* 1979; 43: 857-62.
9. Bauer WC, Igot JP, LeGal Y. Chronologie du cancer mammaire utilisant un modèle de croissance de Gompertz. *ANN Anat Pathol* Paris 1980; 25:39-56
10. Haagensen CD, Bodian C, Haagensen DE. Breast carcinoma — risk and detection. WB Saunders, Philadelphia, 1981.
11. Spratt JS, Heuser LS, Kuhns JG, Greenberg R, Polk HC, Buchanan JB. Variations and associations in histopathology, clinical factors, mammographic patterns and growth rates among breast cancers confirmed in a screened population. In: Mettlin C, Murphy GP, eds. Issues in cancer screening and communications. A Liss, New York, 1982: 295.
12. Fournier D von, Weber E, Hoeffken W, Bauer M, Kubli F, Barth V. Growth rate of 147 mammary carcinomas. *Cancer* 1990; 45: 2198-2207.
13. Baum M. The curability of breast cancer. *Br Med J* 1976; i: 439-42.
14. Fox MS. On diagnosis and treatment of breast cancer. *JAMA* 1979; 241: 489-94.
15. Brinkley D, Haybittle JL. Long-term survival of women with breast cancer. *Lancet* 1984; i: 1118.
16. Le MG, Hill C, Rezvani A, Sarrazin D, Contesso G, Lacour J. Long-term survival of women with breast cancer. *Lancet* 1984: ii: 922.
17. Rutqvist LE, Wallgren A. Long-term survival of 458 young breast cancer patients. *Cancer* 1985; 55: 658-65.
18. Kramer WM, Rush BF. Mammary duct proliferation in the elderly. *Cancer* 1973; 31: 130-37.

19. Nielsen M, Jensen J, Anderson J. Precancerous and cancerous breast lesions during lifetime and at autopsy. *Cancer* 1984: 54: 612- 15.
20. Jackson A. On carcinoma of the breast and its treatment. *Med Press* 1888; i: 552-53.
21. Baum M, Edwards MH. Management of early carcinoma of the breast. *Lancet* 1972; ii: 85.
22. Bruce J. The enigma of breast cancer. *Cancer* 1969; 24: 1314-18.
23. Feinstein AR, Spitz H. The epidemiology of cancer therapy. I. Clinical problems of statistical surveys. *Arch Intern Med* 1969; 123: 171-86.
24. Edelstyn GJA. Surgery and radiotherapy for breast cancer. *Br J Hosp Med* 1969; 3: 1861-72.
25. Lewison EF, Montague ACW, eds. Diagnosis and treatment of breast cancer. Williams & Wilkins, Baltimore, 1981: 3.
26. Canellos GP, Hellman S, Veronesi U. The management of early breast cancer. *N Engl J Med* 1982; 306: 1430- 32.
27. Vorherr H. Adjuvant chemotherapy of breast cancer. Hope — reality — hazard? *Klin Wschr*, 1984; 62: 149-61.
28. Chargaff E. Triviality in science: a brief meditation on fashions. *Perspect Biol Med* 1976; 19: 324-33.
29. Oye RK, Shapiro MF. Reporting results from chemotherapy trials. Does response make a difference in patient survival? *JAMA* 1984; 252: 2722-25.
30. Lee BJ Conservatism in the treatment of primary operable cancer of the breast. In: Report of the international conference on cancer. London. 17-20 July,1928. British Empire Cancer Campaign. J Wright, London, 1928: 131.
31. Fisher B, Bauer M, Margolese R, et al. Five-year results of a randomized clinical trial comparing radical mastectomy and total mastectomy with or without radiation in the treatment of breast cancer. *N Engl J Med.* 1985; 312: 665-73.
32. Fisher B, Redmond C, Fisher ER, et al. Ten-year results of a randomized clinical trial comparing radical mastectomy and total mastectomy with or without radiation. *N Engl J Med.* 1985; 312: 674-81.
33. Goodson WH. The next big question in the treatment of carcinoma of the breast. *Surg Gynecol Obstet* 1983; 356: 795-96.

34. Brinkley D, Haybittle LJ, Houghton J. The Cancer Research Campaign (King's/Cambridge) trial for early breast cancer: an analysis of the radiotherapydata. *Br J Radiol* 1984; 57: 309-16.
35. Park WW, Lees JC. The absolute curability of cancer of the breast. *Surg Gynecol Obstet*; 1951;93: 129-51.
36. Cady B. Lymph node metastases. Indicators, but not governors of survival. *Arch Surg* 1984; 119: 1067-72.
37. Lowe CR. Breast cancer. In: Screening in medical care. Reviewing the evidence. Nuffield Provincial Hospitals Trust. Oxford Univ Press, London, 1968: 33.
38. Wilson RE, Donegan WL, Mettlin C, Natarajan N, Smart CR, Murphy GP. The 1982 national survey of carcinoma of the breast in the United States by American College of Surgeons. *Surg Gynecol Obstet* 1984: 159: 309-18.
39. Faulder C Breast Cancer. Virago Press,Virago, 1982.
40. Frankl G, Ackerman M. Xeromammography and 1200 breast cancers. *Radiol Clin N Am* 1983; 21: 81-91.
41. McKinnon NE. Cancer mortality. The failure of control through case-finding programs. *Surg Gynecol Obstet* 1952; 94: 173-78.
42. Urban JA. Surgical treatment of primary breast cancer — conservative versus radical. In: Lewison EF, Montague ACW, eds. Diagnosis and treatment of breast cancer. Williams & Wilkins, Baltimore, 1981: 119.
43. Urban JA, Papachristou D, Taylor J. Bilateral breast cancer. Biopsy of the opposite breast. *Cancer* 1977; 40: 1968-73.
44. Lynch HT, Harris RE, Organ CH Jr, Lynch JF. Familial indications for prophylactic surgery in breast-cancer-prone families. *Lancet* 1978; i: 265.
45. Slack NH, Nemoto T, Fisher B. Experiences with bilateral primary carcinoma of the breast. *Surg Gynecol Obstet* 1973; 136: 433-40.
46. Chaudary MA, Millis RR, Hoskins EOL, Halder M, Bulbrook RD, Cuzick J, Hayward JL. Bilateral primary breast cancer: a prospective study of disease incidence. *Br J Surg* 1984; 71: 711-14.
47. Betsill WL, Rosen PP, Lieberman PH, Robbins GF. Intraductal carcinoma. Long-term follow-up after treatment by biopsy alone. *JAMA* 1978; 239: 1863-67.

48. Cunningham L. Mastectomy for so-called tubular carcinoma-in-situ. *Lancet* 1980, i: 306.
49. Baum M. Scientific empiricism and clinical medicine. *J R Soc Med* 1981;74: 504-09.
50. Kardinal CG, Yarbro JW. A conceptual history of cancer. *Seminars Oncol* 1979; 4: 396-408.
51. Dodd GD. Present status of thermography, ultrasound and mammography in breast cancer detection. *Cancer* 1977; 39. 2796-805.
52. Roberts CJ, Farrow SC, Charny MC. How much can the NHS afford to spend to save a life or avoid a severe disability? *Lancet* 1985; i: 89-91.
53. Miller AB, Bullbrook RD. Screening. detection and diagnosis of breast cancer. *Lancet* 1982 i:1109-11.
54. Thier SO. Breast-cancer screening: a view from outside the controversy. *N Engl J Med* 1977; 237: 1063-65.
55. Editorial. Early diagnosis and survival in breast cancer. *Lancet* 1981; ii: 785-86.
56. Strax P. Mass screening for control of breast cancer. *Cancer* 1984; 53: 665-70.
57. Mahoney LJ, Bird BL, Cooke GM. Annual clinical examination. The best available screening test for breast cancer.
N Engl J Med 1979; 301: 315-16.
58. Haagensen CD, Asch T. Mammography in medical practice In: Haagensen CD, Bodian C, Haagensen DE, eds. Breast carcinoma — risk and detection. Philadelphia, WB Saunders, 1981: 483.
59. Buttlar CA, Templeton AC. The size of breast masses at presentation. The impact of prior medical training. *Cancer* 1983; 51: 1750-53.
60. Smart CR, Beahrs OH. Breast cancer screening results as viewed by the clinicians. *Cancer* 1979; 43: 851-56.
61. Baker LH. Breast cancer detection demonstration project: five-year summary report. *CA — Cancer J Clinicians* 1982; 32: 194-225.
62. Shapiro S, Strax P, Venet L. Periodic breast cancer screening in reducing mortality from breast cancer. *JAMA* 1971; 215: 1777-85.
63. Kopans DB, Meyer JE, Sadowsky N. Breast imaging.
N Engl J Med 1984; 310: 960-67.

64. Garwin JL. Survival rate calculated from date of diagnosis. *N Engl J Med* 1975; 293: 1045.
65. Moore FD. Breast self-examination. *N Engl J Med* 1978; 299: 305.
66. Turner J, Blaney R, Roy D, Odling-Smee W, Irwin O, Mackenzie G. Does a booklet of breast self-examination improve subsequent detection rates? *Lancet* 1984; ii: 337-39.
67. Philip J, Harris WG, Flaherty C, Joslin CAF, Rustage JH, Wijesinghe DP. Breast self-examination: clinical results from a population-based prospective study. *Br J Cancer* 1984; 50: 7-12.
68. Reimann SP, Safford FH. Statistical study of the interval between discovery and consultation in mammary carcinomas. In: Report of the international conference on cancer. London 17-20 July, 1928. British Empire Cancer Campaign. Wright, London, 1928: 562.
69. Fentiman IS, Cuzick J, Millis RR, Hayward JL. Which patients are cured of breast cancer? *Br Med J* 1984; 289: 1108-11.
70. Carbone PP. A lesson from the mammography issue. *Ann Intern Med* 1978; 88: 703-04.
71. Bailar JC. Mammography: a contrary view. *Ann Intern Med* 1976; 84: 77-84.
72. Bailar JC. Screening for early breast cancer: pros and cons. *Cancer* 1977; 39: 2783-95.
73. Massachusetts Department of Public Health. Mammography — a question. *N Engl J Med* 1976; 294: 395-96.
74. Greenberg DS. X-ray mammography — background to a decision. *N Engl J Med* 1976; 295: 739-40.
75. Fox SH, Moskowitz M, Sanger EI, Kereiakes JG, Milbrath J, Goodman MW. Benefit/risk analysis of aggressive mammographic screening. *Radiology* 1978; 128: 359-65.
76. Morgan RH. Benefit-risk ratios in mammography. In: Lewiston EF, Montague ACW, eds. Diagnosis and treatment of breast cancer. Williams and Wilkins, Baltimore, 1981: 39.
77. Fitzgerald M. Radiation hazards of breast screening. *Br J Radiol* 1983; 56: 283-94.
78. Russell JGB. How dangerous are diagnostic X-rays? *Clin Radiol* 1984; 35: 347-51.

79. Shapiro S. Evidence on screening for breast cancer from a randomized trial. *Cancer* 1977; 39: 2772-82.
80. Knox EG. Simulation studies of breast cancer screening programmes. In: McLachlan G, ed. Probes for health. Nuffield Provincial Hospitals Trust. Oxford University Press, London, 1975:15.
81. Tabar L, Fagerberg CJG, Gad A, et al. Reduction in mortality from breast cancer after mass screening with mammography. Randomised trial from the breast cancer screening working group of the Swedish National Board of Health and Welfare. *Lancet* 1985; i: 829-32.
82. Verbeek ALM, Hendriks JHCL, Holland R, Mravunac M, Sturmans F, Day NE. Reduction of breast cancer mortality through mass screening with modern mammography. First results of the Nijmegen project 1975-1981. *Lancet* 1984; i: 1222-24.
83. Collette HJA, Day NE, Rombach JJ, de Waard F. Evaluation of screening for breast cancer in a non-randomised study (the DOM project) by means of a case-control study. *Lancet* 1984; i: 1224-26.
84. Baum M, McRae KD. Screening for breast cancer. *Lancet* 1984; ii: 462.
85. Roberts MM, Alexander FE, Anderson TJ, et al. The Edinburgh randomised trial of screening for breast cancer: Description of method. *Br J Cancer* 1984; 56: 1-6.
86. Kelley JL, Thieme ET. Impact of public education about cancer on detection and treatment of cancer of the breast by surgery. *Cancer* 1967; 20: 260-62.
87. Leathar DS, Roberts MM. Older women's attitudes towards breast cancer self-examination, and screening facilities: implications for communication. *Br Med J* 1985; 290: 468-70.
88. Maguire GP. Possible psychiatric complications of screening for breast cancer. *Br J Radiol* 1983; 56: 284.
89. Gyllensköid K, Buckau B. A follow-up study of discussion in small groups about education in breast self-examination. Unpublished.
90. Kalache A, Roberts M, Stratton I. Breast cancer: views of general practitioners on its detection and treatment. *J Roy Coll Gen Practit* 1994; 34: 250-54.

3

ACUPUNCTURE: PAST, PRESENT, AND FUTURE

"A chief obstacle in the way of scientific investigation of [this phenomenon] is the difficulty of finding any solid footing in the quagmire of error, self-delusion, and downright imposture ... even in the hands of medical men of high character the proportion of truth to mere error is as Falstaff's halfpenny worth of bread to his intolerable deal of sack." Thus spoke a discerning hypnotist in the heyday of hypnotism nearly a hundred years ago.[1] The same holds good for present-day acupuncture.[2]

Reading through a representative selection of about four hundred articles and two dozen books of the acupuncture literature, I have found that the bulk of it consists of writings by converts, impervious to any criticism, who preach a hermetic doctrine in their own esoteric jargon, liberally peppered with Chinese words. Naturally, financial spoils of a fashionable cure also attract swarms of shady operators and unscrupulous opportunists, who rarely bother to go to print. A minority of acupuncture practitioners, mainly those with medical degrees, are anxious to maintain a link with the main body of the medical profession; they try, often successfully, to present acupuncture to their uninitiated colleagues in a matter-of-fact way as a valuable contribution to the therapeutic armamentarium of orthodox medicine; they use moderate language and the terms of modern medicine. This critical review is mainly concerned with the arguments of these apologists.

I see little point in arguing against patent absurdities, e.g., that acupuncture cures acute bacillary dysentery, that it is effective in

---

From Douglas Stalker and Clark Glymour, *Examining Holistic Medicine*, pp 181-196 (Amherst, NY: Prometheus Books) Copyright 1989. Reprinted by permission of the publisher.

controlling fever, or that it enhances "antiphlogistic[!] ... antishock, and antiparalytic abilities of the body," or that it is of value in the treatment of conjunctivitis, central retinitis, myopia, and cataract - miracles that have the imprimatur of the World Health Organisation (WHO).[3]

The history of acupuncture

The ancient origins of acupuncture are regularly used by the acupuncture apologists as evidence for its intrinsic value. If it is realized that there has been no conceptual development in the theory of acupuncture for the last two thousand years, its antiquity is also its undoing. Lu and Needham[4] have provided a scholarly exposition of the history of acupuncture, and it is a pity that their book is marred by an uncritical acceptance of pseudoscientific claims made by modern acupuncturists, and the text is replete with the marvels of acupuncture hagiography. The attitude of the authors can be judged from a naive admission of one of them who witnessed "her mother's cholera in 1909 surmounting the crisis by the aid of acupuncture." The free mix of fantasy and historical facts in this authoritative book is a trap for the unwary.

In its early stages (the third to the first centuries B.C.), acupuncture was used as a form of bloodletting in a magico-religious ritual during which the malevolent spirit of disease was allowed to escape. The humoral concept was soon replaced by the concept of vital energy (*pneuma*, *Qi*).

Qi is said to flow in channels beneath the surface of the body. The surface markings of these channels are known as "meridians." The acupuncture points (acupoints) are located along these meridians in sites where the *Qi* channels can be directly tapped by the needle. Originally there were 365 such points, corresponding to the days of the year: the human microcosm mirroring cosmic time. The stimulation of acupoints may not only release an excess of *Qi*, but also correct a deficiency, thus maintaining harmony between the opposing metaphysical principles of Yin and Yang.[5]

The only development in the last two millenia has been a gradual increase in acupoints, which now exceed two thousand. (This proliferation has been skilfully exploited by the acupuncture apologists to obfuscate negative results from controlled trials — since any random point is more likely than not to be an acupoint, "the impossibility of choosing placebo points" precludes the possibility of objective evaluation of acupuncture![6])

Acupuncture reached Europe in the seventeenth century and has since been rejected, rediscovered, and forgotten again in four major waves.[7] In the last two decades of that century, acupuncture was fairly well established in Europe, though many physicians, including Thomas Sydenham, were skeptical.[8] Several prominent French physicians and surgeons (Dujardin, Vicq-d'Azyr, Berlioz, Cloquet) advocated acupuncture in the eighteenth and nineteenth centuries, but other, equally prominent doctors were not impressed. For example, Trousseau and Pidoux in their *Traité de Thérapeutique* (1836) accused Dr. Louis Berlioz (the father of the composer) of resurrecting an absurd doctrine from well-deserved oblivion.[9] Electroacupuncture, so popular today, was first used by Sarlandière before 1825.[10] Soulie de Morant, a French diplomat in China, fascinated by acupuncture as a cure for cholera, published his influential book *L'Acupunture Chinoise* in 1939.

While France and Germany were the principal European countries under the spell of acupuncture, periodic upsurges were also noticeable in nineteenth century England. In 1829, the editor of Medico-Chirurgical Review wrote: "A little while ago the town rang with 'acupuncture,' every body talked of it, every one was curing incurable diseases with it; but now not a syllable is said upon the subject."[11] In 1871, Teale quoted a friend from Birmingham: "We used to stick half-a-dozen needles into the deltoid ... with sometimes 'wonderful' results."[12] There were many other enthusiastic reports.[13]

Much of this needling was practised by doctors who had no knowledge of Chinese acupuncture, but results were equally spectacular among believers. Needling the "trigger" points in painful musculoskeletal disorders was found to be beneficial. This so-called "needle effect" was rediscovered recently but it has received little attention, presumably because it is devoid of Oriental mystique.[14]

It is ironic that while Europeans were flirting with needles, the Chinese banned acupuncture, first in 1822, and then a number of times later, the last rejection being issued by the Kuomintang government in 1929. The fate of acupuncture was similar in Japan, where the practice was officially prohibited in 1876. What was the reason for this change in attitude toward a practice revered for thousands of years? Lu and Needham, unwilling to accept the possibility that acupuncture is of little use, tried to explain this sudden devaluation of acupuncture by "a strange Victorian prudery" of the ultra-Confucian moralists.[15] The truth seems to be more prosaic, and grains of it can be found in the Chinese Communist rhetoric: "trampling upon the cultural legacy" and "the cultural aggression" of Western imperialists in nineteenth-century China means, among other things, the introduction of Western medical knowledge, including vaccination; the teaching of anatomy, surgery, anaesthesia; and autopsies.[16]

Huard and Wong cite from a note written in the nineteenth century by some Chinese doctors who had just witnessed an autopsy on two English sailors: "We are overcome by your kindness but everything we have just seen is in complete disagreement with the teaching of our books."[17]

After the victory of the Communists in 1949, acupuncture, together with other forms of traditional Chinese medicine, was revived on Mao's orders. It was a pragmatic political solution to the problem of providing health care for a population of over half a billion, when there were only twenty to thirty thousand doctors who had been trained in Western medicine and who looked mainly after the rich and foreign clientele in cities.[18]

The first European echo of this revival was heard in the Soviet Union, following the return of Soviet doctors from China where they attended courses in *chen-chiou* therapy (acupuncture and moxa) in 1956-1957.[19] However, after the break in political relations, acupuncture publications in the Soviet Union and its satellites tapered off. The strongest official rejection of acupuncture in the Soviet sphere of influence came from the Academy of Sciences of the German Democratic Republic.[20] Enthusiastic reports from Eastern Europe in the 1960s did not go unnoticed in the West,[21] but the Western acupuncturists in general kept a low profile until after Nixon's visit to China in 1972.

Acupuncture "anaesthesia"

In 1958, during the Great Leap Forward, the Chinese invented acupuncture anaesthesia, and by the time the Western cultural and scientific delegations started arriving, the scene was set for breathtaking spectacles of patients operated upon without any anaesthetic, who were smiling, sucking mandarin oranges, and chatting with the delegates, while their brain tumors, goitres, lungs, or stomachs were being removed. The delegations were provided with propaganda material, films, and souvenir needles to take home with them. A typical scene was described by one of the flabbergasted Western observers who witnessed a thyroid adenoma being removed from a Chinese patient: "The patient sat up, had a glass of milk, held up his little red book, and said in a firm voice: 'Long live Chairman Mao and welcome American doctors.' He then put on his pajama top, stepped to the floor and walked out of the operating room."[22]

The same scene is described in Chinese propaganda booklets: "The smiling Hu Shu-hsuan sat up on the operating table and, facing a portrait of Chairman Mao, cheered, 'Long live Chairman Mao!' "[23] Curiously, many Western observers have been adamant that acupuncture has nothing to do with hypnosis, suggestion, or brainwashing.

Compare these stories with an account of an American patient undergoing thyroidectomy under hypnoanalgesia in 1956: "The patient talked amiably to the surgical team throughout the surgery, had a glass of water immediately after the operation, jumped off the table. . . ."[24] Such reports were ignored because hypnosis was old hat, whereas Chinese acupuncture created a stir because it was a novelty for many.

Windsor recalled how on one occasion in 1973 in Beijing (Peking) he performed a pulmonary lobectomy on a young man, who, on being shown the excised tissue, clapped his hands, and after the operation was over, sat up, shook hands with everybody, lifted his tubes and bottles, and walked out.[25] (What was in the bottles?) Close reading of such "eyewitness" reports reveals important pieces of information. The patients were carefully selected, indoctrinated, underwent "ideological preparation," and moreover, they were given premedication, local anaesthetic for skin incision, and parenteral analgesia during the operation, *in addition to* acupuncture.

The credulous acceptance of the Chinese propaganda extolling the merits of acupuncture analgesia (used in "ninety percent" of operations; effective in "ninety-eight percent" of patients) and the parroting of such claims by "eyewitnesses" reminds me of some reports by the Western visitors at the purge trials in the Soviet Union in the 1930s — in their eyes the admission of guilt by the victim was "genuine."

Bonica calculated that even during the zenith of acupuncture anaesthesia in China, it was used in no more than 5 percent of operations,[26] or "more like 1% or 2%."[27] Nevertheless, following meetings between Nixon's personal physician (who was one of the eyewitnesses) and the director of the National Institutes of Health (NIH), a special committee was set up and funds provided to investigate this wonder.[28] The will to believe was stronger than the willingness to pause and think. "Highly respected scientists, though well-meaning, did not have the expertise to critically evaluate their observations."[29]

It has been known for a long time that, with or without hypnosis, some patients can be operated upon without anaesthesia and find the pain is tolerable. Intensity of pain is not directly related to the nature or extent of the wound, but strongly depends on the mental state of the patient and on what pain means to the patient.[30] Mesmerism had been used for surgical operations in England since 1837 and was intensely studied by Elliotson, who was also interested in acupuncture. In France, another acupuncturist, Jules Cloquet, carried out mastectomies on hypnotized patients. Esdaile made a reputation by operating on mesmerized patients in India.[31]

Formal hypnosis, however, is not necessary. Parker operated on many patients in China without any anaesthesia (or acupuncture) and was astonished by their apparent insensibility to pain. In 1843, he performed a mastectomy on a patient, who, when the operation was over, "raised herself from the table without assistance, jumped upon the floor and made her bow to the gentlemen present, in the Chinese style, and walked into another room as though nothing had occurred."[32] Similar observations were made by other Western surgeons in China, such as Lockhart, McPherson, and others. "The manner in which they bear the pain of an operation is perfectly astounding," wrote Gordon in 1863, "a large proportion of those upon whom operations were performed had no chloroform ... some did not even clench their hands or teeth, but lay upon the table perfectly motionless, while their muscles were being cut by the knife and their bones divided by the saw."[33] In Europe, doctors had similar experiences. Lennander published a series of articles describing major operations being carried out painlessly with local anaesthesia only. Mitchell (1907) performed limb amputations, thyroidectomies, mastectomies, and other major surgery without general anaesthesia.[34]

When I read Dimond's paper 1 was reminded of a French soldier who cried "Vive la Nation!" when his leg, in which a huge Prussian ball had lodged, was amputated without anaesthetic in 1793.[35]

One of the operations believed to be particularly suitable for acupuncture anaesthesia is thyroidectomy.[36] In Berne before 1898, Theodor Kocher carried out 1600 thyroidectomies: "The danger in complicated cases has been diminished since general anaesthesia was abandoned. An injection of 1% solution of cocaine is made for the skin incision and intelligent patients, after this has been made painless, bear the remainder of the operation without difficulty."[37] Professor H. E. Ackerknecht kindly brought to my notice a letter by Harvey Cushing written in 1900 in which Cushing expressed his utter astonishment on seeing César Roux operating on goitres in Valois peasants with no anaesthesia.

The Chinese inventors of acupuncture anaesthesia used initially more than fifty needles, but the number gradually dropped to one or two. Would the same effect be achieved with no needles whatsoever? Those who dared to ask such awkward questions were branded as "counter-revolutionary revisionists."[38]

The widely quoted figure of "ninety percent" effectiveness of acupuncture anaesthesia must be seen in the context of the meaning of the word "success" in Chinese propaganda: Grade I ("excellent" — 30 percent of patients), Grade II ("good" — 30 percent of patients), and Grade III ("fair" — 30 percent of patients) comprise "success." In Grade IV the operation has to be abandoned or a general anaesthesia used. To get a glimpse of what this scale actually means, I shall cite from a recent report, published in a reputable journal, on women who were sterilized under local anaesthesia and acupuncture anaesthesia: patients in Grade II were "moaning and groaning," and in Grade III "struggling and otherwise interfering with the operation."[39] Success? Yes, the authors concluded that the method was simple, safe, and economical!

When Bonica asked two Chinese doctors (a surgeon and an anaesthetist) whether they themselves, if undergoing a hernia repair, would choose acupuncture anaesthesia, the virtues of which they were extolling, both expressed a preference for chemical anaesthesia.[40] The lie of acupuncture anaesthesia was exposed in the Chinese press more recently.[41]

The doyen of the British acupuncturists, Felix Mann, found that acupuncture would be "just adequate" for surgery in only ten out of one hundred patients. He used electroacupuncture and the pain of stimulation itself was "so severe that, even though lying horizontally, the patients sometimes feel that they are almost fainting. Interestingly, despite this severe pain, they can carry on an animated conversation and even smile."[42] (I suspect that they could suck an orange as well.) Mann thought that "even if it is unintentional, something allied to hypnosis may be taking place." Other Western experimenters fared no better. Wallis et al. reported that none of their twenty-one obstetric patients obtained adequate analgesia by means of acupuncture. Even in China the anaesthesia could not be adequate since a special fast-cutting technique ("the method of flying knives") had to be developed to minimize the pain of skin incisions.

The acupuncture apologists believe that reports on acupuncture anaesthesia in animals are clear proof that there is something more to it than hypnosis, since animals cannot be influenced by words or political propaganda. They ignore the extensive literature on animal "hypnosis" or "still reaction." Animals undergoing operations under acupuncture anaesthesia have to be tied down firmly[44] —the fear and restraint induce anaesthesia.[45] Acupuncture alone does not produce significant changes in pain tolerance in animals, but pain tolerance is increased in frightened, restrained animals, or in animals in the immobility-reflex-like state.[46]

Critical studies of acupuncture in man

Acupuncture does not induce physiological analgesia since sensory discrimination remains unimpaired. However, the psychological attitude of subjects undergoing acupuncture makes them more reluctant to report pain.[47] Dey et al., in a well-controlled study, failed to demonstrate any effect of acupuncture on pain perception or on galvanic skin responses.[48] Li et al. found acupuncture inferior to hypnosis; acupuncture did not increase pain tolerance.[49] Levine et al. found that in chronic pain, acupuncture was more likely to be effective in patients with high scores for anxiety and depression.[50]

The dissociation of pain perception and pain reporting was documented by Modell et al. in a patient who had undergone augmentation mammoplasty (breast enlargement through plastic surgery) under acupuncture anaesthesia: she found that the skin incision "really hurt" and that cauterization felt as if she were "being touched with a soldering iron." Yet, she did not complain during the operation and two anaesthetists who watched her did not detect any evidence of pain.[51]

What was believed to be the "stoicism" of Chinese patients in the face of pain was their conditioning and not a racial reaction. Knox et al.

found no difference in response to pain (with or without acupuncture) between Oriental subjects and North American subjects.[52]

The complexity of pain perception and the difficulty of separating the psychological from the physiological components are the main reasons for the persistence of irrational beliefs in acupuncture. In disorders in which changes in pathophysiology can be objectively determined, "acupuncture and its theories have long been recognized for the crass unmitigated nonsense they are."[53] Critical observers, however, also find acupuncture useless in painful conditions. Sweet summarized his experience of the value of acupuncture in trigeminal neuralgia (painful spasms of the fifth cranial nerve): in only 9 out of 97 patients treated with acupuncture was there any temporary amelioration of pain, while 6 other patients were sure they got worse.[54] In another study of 100 patients with chronic pain, long-lasting relief was reported by 3 patients, though none of them had reduced their intake of analgesics![55]

The leading British acupuncturist, George T. Lewith, suggested in an editorial in the *British Medical Journal* that objective scientific studies of acupuncture would require a relatively small number of patients since the "predicted" response rates for acupuncture and placebo differ widely — 60 percent and 30 percent, respectively.[56] This belief is shared by the pain expert Melzack.[57] This is a fundamental misunderstanding of placebo. Placebo response can range from 0 percent to 100 percent, depending on circumstances.[58] Even in the studies cited by Lewith, the placebo response varied from 0 percent to 70 percent. The average response of 30 percent applies to ordinary placebos. It is well known that the placebo response to new "therapies" is initially of the order 70 to 90 percent in the enthusiasts' reports and gradually decreases to a 30 to 40 percent baseline in reports of the skeptics.[59] This is why Trousseau advised the medical tyros that they should treat as many patients as possible with the new drug while it still has the power to heal. The Chinese figures of 99 percent success of acupuncture in various disorders[60] are fictional and on a par with election results in totalitarian countries.

In his editorial, Lewith misinformed his readers when he suggested that "the results [of controlled trials] give an overall impression that acupuncture has an analgesic effect in about 60% of patients." This is wishful thinking. The studies in question can be divided into two groups: (1) major studies published in journals of high repute, showing no difference whatsoever between acupuncture and placebo; and (2) observations in lesser-known journals or in acupuncture periodicals, claiming up to 100 percent effectiveness for acupuncture. Surely it is unjustifiable and meaningless to pool the results of these two groups in order to obtain the 60 percent mean.

It has been shown in many studies that acupuncture points are nonspecific and that the same results can be obtained by inserting needles in other sites, not listed in acupuncture atlases.[61] In chronic pain, controlled studies showed that acupuncture was no better than conventional therapy or placebo.[62]

Homuncular acupuncture

What has been said about acupuncture in general holds true also for the many acupuncture variants, such as moxibustion (burning cones of powderized dried leaves over acupoints), acupressure (pressure over acupoints), homeoacupuncture (injection of homeopathic solutions into acupoints), and others. The most popular variant of acupuncture is auricular acupuncture, based on a bizarre notion that the human external ear corresponds point by point to the inner organs and functions of the human body. This is represented by drawings of an inverted homunculus (the body in dwarf form) snugly fitting within the outline of the pinna (outer ear). (Similar representations of the body within the nose, face, hand, or foot have also been described and used for "treatment.") I mention auricular acupuncture only because this mediaeval lunacy occasionally creeps into reputable medical journals[63] and books.[64] The main difficulty with ear acupuncture is that the French homunculus and the Chinese homunculus are markedly different[65] so that the organ allegedly stimulated from the ear will change with the change of the homuncular map used.

The American Journal of Medicine recently published a paper[66] purporting to show that auricular acupuncture is effective against smoking addiction. The reason for publishing this paper by a reputable journal remains obscure. The study was uncontrolled and the patients were subjected to antismoking indoctrination *in addition to* acupuncture. The authors discovered the "antismoking" ear point by chance when two overweight nurses were treated for obesity by a needle in the ear and suddenly stopped smoking. If the "antiobesity" point was identical with the "antismoking" point, one would expect that overweight smokers thus treated would lose weight. No data on weight loss were given in the 514 patients studied. (The effectiveness in the treatment of obesity was such that one patient was said to have lost six pounds over a weekend!) The authors claimed a success rate of 88 percent. Of 514 patients presented for treatment only 339 were "evaluable." Of these 339 self-selected patients, 297 stopped smoking after four weeks (this is the 88 percent) but we were not told how many of them relapsed, because only 220 patients were "available" at a follow-up; of these, 31 percent had resumed smoking. Thus, the total of patients who resumed smoking, assuming that those lost or excluded also resumed smoking, would be 362, i.e., 70 percent treatment failure. Controlled studies showing that acupuncture for smokers is no better than indoctrination were not cited.[67] Editors of medical journals should be particularly vigilant when dealing with such partisan reports.

The endorphin hypothesis

Following conflicting reports that the opiate antagonist naloxone abolished acupuncture analgesia,[68] it has become a new dogma of acupuncturists that acupuncture analgesia is mediated by endogenous opiates (endorphins). The endorphin hypothesis has brought acupuncturists and biological psychiatrists together. The latter believe that an imbalance of endorphins is a cause of mental disease and could be corrected by bloodletting.[69] The endorphin theory of mental disease is modelled on the Yin-Yang doctrine, and acupuncture has been used for treatment of mental disease both in China and the United States.[70] Recently *The Lancet* published an acupuncture article in which it was claimed that acupuncture improved chronic pain *and* psychiatric symptoms. The study was uncontrolled and the difference in the mean pain score was only 26 percent, based on self-reporting by patients "experiencing serious psychiatric difficulties."[71]

The endorphin "explanation" of acupuncture has put the cart firmly before the horse. Two simple questions would have to be asked and then answered before appealing to endorphins. First, do endorphins correlate with clinical pain? Second, does acupuncture release endorphins?

There is no good evidence that acupuncture-induced pain relief is mediated by endorphin release.[72] There is no correlation between plasma endorphin levels and pain; even patients with β-endorphin levels 300-600 times the normal had no impairment of sensitivity to pain.[73] Intravenous injections of β-endorphin have no analgesic effect in man.[74] Studies usually quoted by acupuncture apologists in support of acupuncture-induced release of endorphins are either inapplicable to acupuncture in humans (e.g., electrostimulation of brain areas in animals) or conflicting.[75]

The endorphin hypothesis has also been repeatedly invoked in the use of acupuncture as a treatment for opiate addiction. This "treatment" was based on uncontrolled or seriously suspect studies. Gossop et al. found that acupuncture failed to suppress withdrawal symptoms and was markedly inferior to methadone treatment. Several addicts found no difference between the use of acupuncture and withdrawing "cold turkey"(a sudden opiate withdrawal).[76]

It appeared for a time that the endorphin hypothesis could salvage acupuncture, even if acupuncture were a form of placebo, since placebo itself might be mediated by endorphins. This hope was shattered by experiments conducted by Gracely et al., who demonstrated that naloxone does not antagonize the placebo.[77]

While many acupuncturists are gradually coming to terms with the weakness of the endorphin hypothesis, the possible speculations on the humoral (fluid) basis of acupuncture, originating mainly from Communist China, are endless, though of no clinical significance.[78]

Why does acupuncture work?

There is no denying that acupuncture is effective in some patients with functional and psychosomatic disorders. So is placebo. It is also a fact that the acupuncture effect is unpredictable and unreliable. Results depend on the faith. "Negative findings . . . may reflect negative attitudes on the part of the experimental subject."[79]

The simple explanation for a better average response to acupuncture than to more conventional placebos is its very unconventionality, the mystique surrounding an ancient Oriental ritual, and the magic of model mannikins and golden needles. Once these trappings are removed and the veil of the mystery lifted, acupuncture will again be relegated to its original place among counter-irritants,[80] such as cupping, sinapisms (mustard plasters), bee stings, vesicants, cautery (moxa). and setons (known in the modem acupuncture terminology as "thread acupuncture"), or more recently, vibration, electrostimulation, and temperature changes.[81] By discussing acupuncture in terms of placebo, distraction, suggestion, and hypnosis, and taking into account the natural history of self-limiting and functional disorders that acupuncture is supposed to cure, it will lose its attraction, its novelty, and its power over the mind of the gullible.

The gullible include scientists. A plea for investigation of acupuncture was made by a medical historian: "No matter how bizarre a therapy is, how lacking in rationale, and how uncertain its value, it is concerned with patients and hence it is a phenomenon which must interest the world of medicine."[82] While skeptical inquiry is safer than an outright dogmatic rejection, it is disheartening to see serious scientists conducting incompetent investigations. To use an analogy from parapsychology: scientists did not find the explanation of the Uri Geller phenomenon by studying bent spoons under the microscope; they found the answer by studying Uri Geller himself. The question was not how the spoon bent, but how Geller made the scientists believe that it bent on its own. Similarly, when studying the phenomenon of acupuncture, the minute biochemical analysis and the search for endorphins in acupunctured subjects is misdirected, since the problem is not biochemical but psychological and cultural. Just as a student of the Geller "mental" bending would be well advised to consult a professional magician, so a student of acupuncture will profit from the expert advice of a stage hypnotist.

Kroger, who is experienced in hypnoanalgesia, pointed out the similarities between acupuncture and hypnosis: conditioning, ritual indoctrination, autogenic training, misdirection, autosuggestion.[83] In China, the strong traditional belief in the power of needles was further augmented by sociopolitical rewards for good behaviour during acupuncture. Kroger knew from his experience that scientists unfamiliar with the phenomena of suggestion and autohypnosis would not believe that the patient is hypnotized without a formal induction and without falling asleep.

For obvious reasons, the possibility of hypnosis or suggestion is strongly resisted by acupuncture apologists. They even twist the evidence. For example, Lewith commented on a study of Moore and Berk[84] as follows: "They demonstrated that suggestibility did not affect the outcome in their study." Yet Moore and Berk wrote: "The average improvement in discomfort scores, as well as the percentage of those who achieved 60% or more relief increased with hypnotic susceptibility [from 29% to 55%]." "In demonstrating ... a possible link between response to treatment and susceptibility to hypnosis, we are challenging those who believe that acupuncture offers a unique approach to pain control."

Chaves and Barber suggested six tentative headings under which acupuncture anaesthesia could be investigated: (1) strong belief, (2) concomitant use of other analgesia, (3) overestimation of surgical pain, (4) distraction produced by needles, (5) special preparation and indoctrination, (6) suggestion.[85] Excluding points 2 and 3, the headings are equally applicable for other acupuncture treatments.

The future of acupuncture

In the last few years the gap between acupuncture practitioners and rational medicine has widened and will continue to do so. In the keynote address at the founding convention of the American Association of Acupuncturists and Oriental Medicine in Los Angeles in 1981, R.A. Dale announced the coming of the great age of holistic harmony in which acupuncture will play a pivotal role. Since his remarks represent the mainstream of acupuncture ideology, they are worth our attention: "Acupuncture is a part of a larger struggle going on today between the old and the new, between dying and rebirthing, between the very decay and death of our species and our fullest liberation. Acupuncture is part of a New Age which facilitates integral health and the flowering of our humanity."[88]

Dale differentiated five attitudes of the medical profession to acupuncture: (1) "the reactionary extreme," which should be ignored, isolated, and exposed; (2) "the conservative opposition," which should be supplied with data and statistics ("although the American Medical Association will not be convinced by such arguments, some of its members will be"); (3) "the liberal support," whose members are "usually cautious not to discuss their views with their colleagues from Groups 1 and 2," but they are "excellent candidates" for Group 4, "the progressive support"; (5) "support by medical heretics," who are "excellent candidates not only for active membership in our association but for leadership roles."

The tactic and strategy to be adopted by the acupuncturists when dealing with the public are, according to Dale's advice, as follows: (1) undermine their faith in modern medicine and science, (2) educate them in their need for alternative medicine, and (3) explain to them that what they need is not a medical specialist but an acupuncture generalist.

The openness of this document is disarming. Let us note, however, that

Dale's "New Age" is matched only by the WHO's messianic rhetoric of "health for all by the year of 2000." Unreal promises and false hopes raised by the medical profession, no less irrational than the illusions of "alternative" medicine, deserve to be criticized as mercilessly as the deceptive fancies and will-o'-the-wisps of the holistic prophets and quackupuncturists.

References

1. Hart E. Hypnotism, Mesmerism and the New Witchcraft. 2nd ed. Smith & Elder, London, 1896: 168.

2. Skrabanek P. Acupuncture and the Age of Unreason. *Lancet* 1984; i: 1169-71.

3. Bannerman RH Acupuncture: The WHO View, World Health (December 1979): 24-29.

4. Lu G-D and Needham J. Celestial Lancets: A History and Rationale of Acupuncture and Moxa. Cambridge University Press, London, 1980.

5. Epler DC. Bloodletting in Early Chinese Medicine and its Relation to the Origin of Acupuncture. *Bulletin of the History of Medicine* 54 (1980): 337-367.

6. Liao SJ. Recent Advances in the Understanding of Acupuncture. *Yale Journal of Biology and Medicine* 1978; 51: 55-65.

7. Ackerknecht EH. Zur Geschichte der Akupunktur. *Anaestetist* 1974; 23 : 37-38; Ackerknecht EH. Akupunktur—Gestern, Heute, Morgen. *Schweizerische Aerztezeitung* 1972; 33: 1067-68.

8. Lu and Needham, op. cit., 292.

9. Lacassagne J. Le docteur Louis Berlioz—Introducteur de l'Acupuncture en France. *Presse Médicale* 1954; 62: 1359-60.

10. Anon. *Edinburgh Medical and Surgical Journal* 1827; 27: 190-200; 334-49.

11. Anon. Acupuncturation. *Medico-Chirurgical Review* (London)1829;11: 166-67.

12. Teale TP. On the Relief of Pain and Muscular Disability by Acupuncture. *Lancet* 1871; i: 567-68.

13. Elliotson J. Acupuncture. In Forbes J, Tweedie A, and Connolly J eds. The Cyclopaedia of Practical Medicine. vol. 1. Sherwood, London, 1833: 32-34; Anon. When Acupuncture Came to Britain. (editorial) *British Medical Journal* 1973; 4: 687-88; Lorimer G. Acupuncture and its Application in the Treatment of Certain Forms of Chronic Rheumatism. *British Medical Journal* 1885; 2: 956-58; Anon. Employment of Acupuncture as a Counterirritant. *Practitioner* 1868; 371-72; see also Skrabanek, note 2.

14. Lewit K. The Needle Effect in the Relief of Myofascial Pain. *Pain* 1979; 6 : 83-90; Frost FA, Jessen B, and Siggaard-Andersen J. A Control, Double-blind Comparison of Mepivacaine Injection versus Saline Injection for Myofascial Pain. *Lancet* 1980; i: 499-501.

15. Lu and Needham, op. cit., 160.

16. Huard P. and M. Wong M. Chinese Medicine. Weidenfeld & Nicolson, London, 1968.

17. Ibid., 135.

18. Ibid., 159.

19. Ibid., 150.

20. Anon. Statement Regarding Acupuncture by the Medical Council of the Academy of Sciences of the German Democratic Republic. *Zeitschrift für Experimentelle Chirurgie* 1981; 14: 67. For a critical review of German literature, see Mattig W and Gertier. A. Akupunktur: Scharlatanerie oder therapeutische Bereicherung? *Innere Medizin* 1983; 10: 208-12; 247-52.

21. Veith I. Acupuncture Therapy — Past and Present: Verity or Delusion? *Journal of the American Medical Association* 1962; 180: 478-84.

22. Dimond EG. Acupuncture Anaesthesia: Western Medicine and Chinese Traditional Medicine. *Journal of the American Medical Association* 1971; 218: 1558-63.

23. Anon. Acupuncture Anaesthesia. Foreign Languages Press, Peking, 1972, 9.

24. Kroger WS. Acupunctural Analgesia: Its Explanation by Conditioning Theory, Autogenic Training, and Hypnosis. *American Journal of Psychiatry* 1973; 130: 855-60.

25. Windsor HM. Cardiac Surgery in China. *Medical Journal of Australia* 1984; 1: 599-602.

26. Bonica JJ. Acupuncture Anesthesia in the People's Republic of China: Implications for American Medicine. *Journal of the American Medical Association* 1974; 229 : 1317-25.

27. Murphy TM and Bonica JJ. Acupuncture Analgesia and Anesthesia. *Archives of Surgery* 1977; 112 : 896-902.

28. Culliton BJ. Acupuncture: Fertile Ground for Faddist and Serious NIH Research. *Science* 1972; 177 : 592-94.

29. Murphy and Bonica, note 27 above.

30. Beecher HK. Relationship of Significance of Wound to Pain Experienced. *Journal of the American Medical Association* 1956; 161: 1609-13.

31. Rosen G. Mesmerism and Surgery: A Strange Chapter in the History of Anaesthesia. *Journal of the History of Medicine* 1946 ; 1: 527-50.

32. Johnson DA. History and the Understanding of Acupuncture Anaesthesia. *Southern Medical Journal* 1983; 76:497-98.

33. Ibid.

34. Chaves JF and Barber TX. Acupuncture Analgesia: A Six-factor Theory. In Krippner S ed. Psychoenergetic Systems. Gordon & Breach Science Publishers, New York, 1979, 169-78.

35. Anon. An Incident of Pre-anaesthetic Surgery. *Medical Press* 1890; 2: 239.

36. Cheng SB and Ding LK. Practical Application of Acupuncture Analgesia. *Nature* 1973; 242: 559-60.

37. Anon. 600 More Goitre Operations. *Medical Press* 1908; 2: 624.
38. See note 23.
39. Dias PLR. and Subramanium S. Minilaparotomy Under Acupuncture Analgesia. *Journal of the Royal Society of Medicine* 1984; 77: 295-98.
40. See note 26.
41. Gan X and Tao N. in the Shangai daily *Wen-Hui-Bao* (October 22, 1980).
42. Mann F. Acupuncture Analgesia: Report of 100 Experiments. *British Journal of Anaesthesiology* 1974; 46: 361-64.
43. Wallis L, Shnider SM, Palahniuk RJ and Spivey HT. An Evaluation of Acupuncture Analgesia in Obstetrics. *Anaesthesiology* 1974; 41: 596-601.
44. Macdonald A. Acupuncture: From Ancient Art to Modern Medicine. Allen & Unwin, London, 1982. 126.
45. Kroger, note 24.
46. Galeano C and Leung CY. Has Acupuncture an Analgesic Effect in Rabbits? *Pain* 1978; 4: 265-71; Galeano C, Leung CY, Robitaille R and Roy-Chabot T. Acupuncture Analgesia in Rabbits. *Pain* 1979; 6: 71-81.
47. Clark WC and Yang JC. Acupunctural Analgesia: Evaluation by Signal Detection Theory. *Science* 1975; 184: 1096-98; Clark WC, Yang JC and Hall W. Acupuncture. Pain, and Signal Detection Theory. *Science* 1975; 189: 66-68.
48. Day RL, Kitahata LM, Kao FF, Motoyama EK, and Hardy JD. Evaluation of Acupuncture Anesthesia: A Psychophysical Study. *Anesthesiology.* 1975; 43: 507-17; Day RL. Acupuncture. *Lancet* 1984; ii: 175.
49. Ailberg CLLD, Lansdell H, Gravitz MA, Chen TC, Ting CY, Bak AF and Blessing D. Acupuncture and Hypnosis: Effects on Induced Pain. *Experimental Neurology* 1975; 49: 272-80.
50. Levine JD, Gormley J. and Fields HL. Observations on the Analgesic Effects of Needle Puncture (Acupuncture). *Pain* 1976; 2: 149-59.
51. Modell JH, Lee PKY, Bingham HG, Greer DM and Habal MB. Acupuncture Anaesthesia: A Clinical Study.

Anaesthesia and Analgesia 1976; 55: 508-12.

52. Knox VJ, Shum K and McLaughlin DM. Response to Cold Pressor Pain and to Acupuncture Analgesia in Oriental and Occidental Subjects. *Pain* 1977; 4: 49-57.

53. Sweet WH. Some Current Problems in Pain Research and Therapy (Including Needle Puncture, 'Acupuncture'). *Pain* 1981; 10: 297-309.

54. Ibid.

55. Murphy and Bonica, note 27.

56. Lewith GL. Can We Assess the Effects of Acupuncture? *British Medical Journal* 1984; 288: 1475-76.

57. Melzack R. Acupuncture and Musculoskeletal Pain. *Journal of Rheumatology* 1978; 5:119-20.

58. Anon. Shall I Please? (editorial) *Lancet* 1983; ii: 1465-66.

59. Benson H and McCallie DP. Angina Pectoris and the Placebo Effect. *New England Journal of Medicine* 1979; 300: 1424-28.

60. National Symposia of Acupuncture and Moxibustion and Acupuncture Anaesthesia. Foreign Languages Press, Beijing, 1979; *passim*. Essentials of Chinese Acupuncture. Foreign Languages Press, Beijing, 1980; *passim*.

61. Gaw AC, Chang LW and Shaw L-C. Efficacy of Acupuncture on Osteoarthritic Pain: A Controlled, Double-blind Study. *New England Journal of Medicine* 1975; 293: 375-78; Lee PK, Andersen TW, Modell JH and Saga SA. Treatment of Chronic Pain with Acupuncture. *Journal of the American Medical Association* 1975; 232: 1133-35; Lynn B and Perl ER. Acupuncture Analgesia of the Skin in Relation to the Traditional Meridian Map. *Journal of Physiology (London)* 1975; 245: 83P-85P; Weintraub M, Petursson S, Schwartz M, Barnard T, Morgan JP, Gluckman J. and Geertsma RH. Acupuncture in Musculoskeletal Pain: Methodology and Results in a Double-blind Controlled Clinical Trial. *Clinical Pharmacology and Therapeutics* 1975; 17: 248; Moore MY and Berk SN. Acupuncture for Chronic Shoulder Pain: An Experimental Study with Attention to the Role of Placebo and Hypnotic Susceptibility. *Annals of*

Internal Medicine 1976; 84: 381-84; Edelist G, Gross AE and Langer F. Treatment of Low Back Pain with Acupuncture. *Canadian Anaesthetists' Society Journal* 1976; 23:303-306; Godfrey CM.and Morgan P. A Controlled Trial of the Theory of Acupuncture in Musculoskeletal Pain. *Journal of Rheumatology* 1978; 5: 121-24; Co LL, Schmitz TH, Havdala H, Reyes A and Westerman MP. Acupuncture: An Evaluation in the Painful Crises of Sickle-Cell Anemia, *Pain* 1979; 7; 181-85; Hansen PE, Hansen JH and Bentzen, O. Acupuncture Treatment of Chronic Unilateral Tinnitus: A Double-blind Cross-over Trial. *Clinical Otolaryngology* 1982; 7: 325-329; Chow OKW, So SY, Lam WK, Yu DYC and Yeung CY Effect of Acupuncture on Exercise-induced Asthma. *Lung* 1983; 161: 321-26.

62. Fernandes L, Berry H, Clark RJ, Bloom B and Hamilton EBD. Clinical Study Comparing Acupuncture, Physiotherapy, Injection, and Oral Anti-inflammatory Therapy in Shoulder-cuff Lesions. *Lancet* 1980; i: 208-209; Lewith GT,Field J and Machin D. Acupuncture Compared with Placebo in Post-herpetic Pain. *Pain* 1983; 17: 361-68.

63. Melzack R and Katz J. Auriculotherapy Fails to Relieve Chronic Pain: A Controlled Crossover Study. *Journal of the American Medical Association* 1984; 251: 1041-43; Lewith, GT, Field J and Machin D. Acupuncture Compared with Placebo in Post-herpetic Pain. *Pain* 1983; 17: 361-68; Dang CV. The Ear Lobe Crease, Chromosomes, Acupuncture, and Atherosclerosis. *Lancet* 1984; i: 1083; Choy DSJ, Lutzker L and Meltzer L. Effective Treatment for Smoking Cessation. *American Journal of Medicine* 1983; 75: 1033-36; Oleson TD, Kroening RJ and Bresler DE. An Experimental Evaluation of Auricular Diagnosis: The Somatotopic Mapping of Musculoskeletal Pain at Ear Acupuncture Points. *Pain* 1980;8: 217-29.

64. Lu and Needham, op. cit., 164f.

65. Oleson TD and Kroening RJ. A Comparison of Chinese and Nogier Auricular Acupuncture Points. *American Journal of Acupuncture* 1983; 11: 205-23.

66. Choy DSJ, Lutzker L and Meltzer L. Effective Treatment for Smoking

Cessation. *American Journal of Medicine* 1983; 75: 1033-36.

67. Lamontagne Y, Annable L and Gagnon M-A. Acupuncture for Smokers: Lack of Long-term Therapeutic Effect in a Controlled Study. *Canadian Medical Association Journal* 1980; 122: 787-90.

68. Anon. Endorphins Through the Eye of a Needle? (editorial) *Lancet* 1981;i: 480-82.

69. Skrabanek P. Naloxone in Schizophrenia. *Lancet* 1982; ii: 1270; Skrabanek P. Haemodialysis in Schizophrenia — déjà vu or idée fixé? *Lancet* 1982; i: 1404-1405.

70. Kane J. and Di Scipio WJ. Acupuncture Treatment of Schizophrenia. *American Journal of Psychiatry* 1979; 136: 297-302.

71. Kiser RS, Khatami M, Gatchel RJ, Huang X-Y. Bhatia K and Altshuler KZ. Acupuncture Relief of Chronic Pain Syndrome Correlates with Increased Plasma Met-enkephalin Concentrations. *Lancet* 1983; ii: 1394-96; Skrabanek P. Acupuncture and Endorphins. *Lancet* 1984; i: 220.

72. Anon. Endorphins Through the Eye of a Needle. (editorial) *Lancet* 1981;i: 480-82.

73. Willer JC, Sheng-Shu L, Bertagna X and Girard F. Pituitary β-endorphin Not Involved in Pain Control in Some Pathophysiological Conditions. *Lancet* 1984; ii: 293-96.

74. Hosobuchi U and Li CH. Demonstration of the Analgesic Activity of Human β-endorphin in Six Patients. In Usdin E, Bunney M.E. and Kline N.S. eds. Endorphins in Mental Disease and Research. Macmillan, New York, 1979: 529-34.

75. See note 72.

76. Gossop M, Bradley B, Strang J and Connell P. The Clinical Effectiveness of Electro-stimulation vs. Oral Methadone in Managing Opiate Withdrawal. *British Journal of Psychiatry* 1984; 144: 203-208.

77. Gracely RH, Dubner R, Wolskee P and Deeter WR. Placebo and Naloxone can Alter Postsurgical Pain by Separate Mechanisms. *Nature* 1983; 306: 264-265; Anon. Shall I Please? (editorial) *Lancet* 1983; ii: 1465-66.

78. Han JS and Terenius L. Neurochemical Basis of Acupuncture Analgesia. *Annual Review of Pharmacology and Toxicology* 1982; 22: 193-220.

79. Chapman CR. Psychophysical Evaluation of Acupuncture Analgesia. *Anesthesiology* 1975; 43: 501-503.

80. Williams CJB. Counter-irritation. In Forbes J, Tweedie A and Connolly J eds. The Cyclopaedia of Practical Medicine, vol. 1 Sherwood, London, 1833: 483-92.

81. Gammon GD and Starr I. Studies on the Relief of Pain by Counterirritation. *Journal of Clinical Investigation* 1941; 20: 13-20.

82. See note 21.

83. Kroger WS. Acupunctural Analgesia: Its Explanation by Conditioning Theory, Autogenic Training, and Hypnosis. *American Journal of Psychiatry* 1973; 130: 855-60.

84. Lewith GT. How Effective Is Acupuncture in the Management of Pain? *Journal of the Royal College of General Practitioners* 1984; 34: 275-78; Moore and Berk, see note 61.

85. Chaves JF and Barber TX Acupuncture Analgesia: A Six-factor Theory. In Krippner S ed. Psychoenergetic Systems. Gordon & Breach, New York, 1979: 169-78.

86. Dale RA. The Origins and Future of Acupuncture. *American Journal of Acupuncture* 1982; 10: 101-20.

4

CONVULSIVE THERAPY - A CRITICAL APPRAISAL OF ITS ORIGIN AND VALUE

The subject of electroconvulsive therapy (ECT) has been rarely discussed in a rational, impassive manner; it tends to polarise discussants into the apologists who turn a deaf ear to any criticism and the denouncers who do not bother to acquaint themselves with the facts. This review is an attempt at an impartial and critical assessment of the evidence for the therapeutic value of ECT and the rationale for its use.

The common tendency to disown the origins of modern convulsive therapy and to dissociate it from its past creates new myths and obscures the unchanging empirical basis of the treatment. Historical analysis provides us not only with the sources of instinctive revulsion the anti-ECT activists feel about ECT, but also with the precedents of ECT abuse. Excesses and abuses of ECT, which are bound to occur in the absence of strict ethical guidelines, only supply further ammunition to the campaigners for the abolition of ECT. Analysis of the reasons for ECT abuse is essential if ECT is to survive as a treatment modality with a limited potential in selected cases.

Since ancient times there have been two fundamentally different approaches to the therapy of mental disease: somatotherapy and psychotherapy. This therapeutic dualism betrays persistent uncertainty as to whether mental disease is due to a sick mind or a sick brain. The predilection for one or the other mode of treatment, or for a mixture of both, is determined by the attitude of the therapist to the dichotomy of the mind and the brain. Paradoxically, terror and fear, used in the past as a form of brutal psychotherapy, was invoked by the pioneers of the modern convulsive therapy (a form of somatotherapy) as a possible explanation of its effectiveness.

This paper first appeared in the *Irish Medical Journal*, June 1986, Volume 79, No 6, pages 157-165

Fink, in an attempt to defend the current use of ECT against emotional and uninformed criticism, was at pains to stress that neither electricity, nor "shock", nor convulsions are necessary, since epileptiform brain discharges can be triggered chemically, shock abolished by anaesthesia, and convulsions made invisible by muscle relaxant.[1] While the modified method of administering ECT precludes the patient remembering the procedure and is less upsetting for the attendant staff, the brain is "shocked" in exactly the same way to exactly the same extent. It is only the epiphenomena of the electroshock which have been removed. By modifying ECT, the method has become a part of the armamentarium of biological psychiatry, since the possible psychological effects of the fear of older forms of convulsive therapy have been virtually eliminated. The term electroplexy, recommended by some psychiatrists as a less frightening label, has a euphemistic value only for those who do not know any Greek.

Historical perspective

It has been repeatedly observed and noted that severe psychological or physical shocks can result in recovery from insanity, and the history of psychiatry abounds with weird examples of such treatments. Ackerknecht pointed out that some of the old methods were so drastic that their comparison with 20th century shock therapy is appropriate.[2] Modern convulsive therapy followed in the wake of pyroshock treatment of general paralysis of the insane, and subsequent attempts to treat mental disease with toxic shocks, anaphylactic shocks, transfusion shocks, using injections of metal salts, foreign proteins, infective material, animal blood, etc.[3,4]

It is often said that ECT has proved its usefulness, despite the lack of an acceptable theory as to how it works, as testified by psychiatrists who use it. This amounts to a tautology. The same claims have been made for all the unproven therapies of the past, such as bloodletting, which produced great cures till they were abandoned as useless. It is not long ago since insulin comas, metrazol shocks, and ECT were treatments of choice for schizophrenia. But even the quondam advocates of shock therapy, Sargant and Slater, said about it: "early satisfactory results in schizophrenia, some of them brilliant, have not maintained themselves with time."[5]

The role of terror in treatment

Terror as a therapy for insanity has been used since antiquity. Gaub in *De Regime mentis* (1763) mentions that "chance first taught physicians that a headlong fall into the sea or submersion in water, employed in ancient times against rabies, is of great help against many [mental] diseases", and this has been confirmed by experience. The inhabitants of Lyons showed Borrichius, during his travels in France, a lofty site from which the insane were thrown headlong into the Rhône and repeatedly drawn out on a line in order to teach them sense again, this measure having been adopted for its good results and not as a punishment. Helmolt testifies that with this bold measure the English physician Robertson restored the use of reason to many insane persons. "The entire effect, great as it is, is not in the least due to some peculiar virtue of water, but solely due to the precipitation of the mind into the depth of terror and anguish as a result of the threat of suffocation. What is needed, then, is a machine that will inspire extreme terror, and a submersion of such duration and frequency that life itself is put in hazard and doubt arises when the man is withdrawn whether he is quite dead or can still be revived; otherwise nothing fully effective is to be awaited."[6]

Sudden ducking of patients was abolished by Pinel and Esquirol,[2] but the idea of a beneficial effect of psychological shock and terror in the treatment of insanity has not been abandoned. "It has been the idea for ages that insanity might be cured by sudden shocks, and this belief led in former times to great abuses."[7] "The physical shock has occasionally been known to produce a good moral impression."[8] "In some continental asylums the patients were chained in a well, and the water was allowed gradually to ascend in order to terrify the patient with the prospect of inevitable death."[9] The pit-and-pendulum methods being abandoned, patients were treated with cold-water douches.

Forbes Winslow reviewed a case of death under shower in a pauper patient on whose head 20-40 gallons of water fell every minute for half an hour, and commented with acerbity: "The difficulty will be to persuade the public that the baths were not used as a quasi-punishment."[10] On special rotatory machines used in most British asylums, "instant discharge of the content of the stomach, bowels, and bladder, in quick succession" could be readily achieved.[9]

These examples of terror treatment are more than of historical interest; they form the relevant background for our understanding of the tradition and rationale underlying the introduction of modern convulsive therapy. Many psychiatrists believed (and some of them still do) that the element of fear involved in shock therapies is itself therapeutic. "Psychiatrists repeatedly stated that if a patient is threatened with death and annihilation, all 'imaginary' symptoms will disappear and efforts will be made on the part of the organism to protect itself".[11] The "feeling of horror" before the onset of convulsion after the injection of camphor, metrazol, triazol, picrotoxine, ammonium chloride, and other convulsants, caused a "real dread" of such treatment.[12] "Patients beg not to be treated .... they implore physicians and nurses."[13] "The majority soon grows to fear the injections and a few reach a pitiable state of apprehension and alarm."[14] "It is not altogether excluded that this very anxiety and fear might possibly be just as important as the other phases of the convulsion... The various fears and forebodings inherent in the psychoses become prominent when the patient, is led or dragged into a room where several persons await him..."[11] The "feeling of impending death," "sinking slowly into the hole," "extreme fear" — these are descriptions of patients' reactions used by the advocates of the shock treatment. "The use of cardiazol shocks ... sometimes appear to us to be comparable to an explosive which makes a breach but at the same time may produce damage so far not well defined... We heard our patients objecting violently to the anticipated attack and vainly exerting all their will-power to fight it off."[15]

The patients' views are rarely included in these accounts. One patient was quoted as saying: "They (the injections) make me feel as though a great big policeman was jumping on top of me."[14] Although unmodified ECT was introduced as a humane improvement on the earlier versions of convulsive therapy, patients felt that they were "going to the electric chair," to be "burnt crisp" and to "never wake up."[16] Subsequent modifications introduced new terror: patients given muscle-relaxants without anaesthesia complained bitterly of the terrifying feeling of suffocation and paralysis.[17] Even though the element of terror has been eliminated from the present practice of ECT, many patients are still afraid of it. Freeman and Kendell[18] asked their patients what they thought about modern ECT: 39% thought it was a frightening treatment to have and another 16% did not know (perhaps they did not want to disappoint their psychiatrists). However, it is unlikely that fearful anticipation contributes to the effect of ECT in severely depressed and withdrawn patients.

Dehumanising effect of shock treatment on psychiatrists

Fink admits that the catalogue of the misuses of ECT is depressing, but suggests that it is the abusers and not the instrument which is guilty.[19] This is undoubtedly true. In the same way, surgery should not be blamed for vivisection excesses. Unfortunately, the instrument alone allowing the operator to "zap" the patient by pressing a button tends to dehumanise some of its users.

The layman's reaction to ECT is understandable. Even Cerletti, when his first patient shouted: "Not again: It will kill me!" was frightened and thought that ECT should be abolished,[20,21] though soon later after the novelty of the experience wore off, Cerletti used ECT indiscriminately. Similarly, when Meduna selected his first patient in a state hospital for cardiazol shock and witnessed the effect, his legs gave way, he trembled, was drenched in sweat, and his face turned ashen grey.[22] A few years later he speculated that camphor convulsions, already abandoned because they were preceded by a state of "anxiety and panic associated with assaultive and suicidal behaviour" could be used experimentally on human subjects for "studying the phases of the seizure" because the camphor-induced convulsion develops as in a slow-motion picture.[15] Unfortunately there were "doctors" who did this type of experiment on prisoners. The staff of the Psychiatric Institute at the University of Illinois studied metrazol convulsions in male and female patients who had to undress completely for the procedure. The convulsions of the naked patients were filmed for a further "study" by the "researchers."[13]

Greenblatt recalled how during his training he "was allowed to inject (Metrazol) into chronically ill patients at Worcester State Hospital in Massachusetts against their terrified and frightened resistance, which...was overpowered by several burly attendants."[23]

Dehumanisation is also shown in the language used: "As was our custom with dogs... we fixed the electrodes on the selected patient;"[21] "a convenient mouth gag is provided by a dog's rubber bone."[5] The lack of moral sense in Cerletti's days can be illustrated by the fact that he obtained permission to experiment on pigs in a slaughter-house,[21] but he did not bother to obtain permission to experiment on the first human victim.

Levenson and Willett discussed unconscious attitudes of therapists about ECT, which include the fantasy of omnipotence, and the fantasy of killing and resurrecting the patient; they pointed out that "ECT may seem like an overwhelming assault or a sexual act, which may resonate with the therapist's aggressive and libidinal conflicts."[24]

Following the memorandum on ECT by the Royal College of Psychiatrists,[25] the editor of The British Journal of Psychiatry accused a consultant of being "inhumane" in administering ECT without asking the patient or the relatives.[26] A few years later, Pippard and Ellam showed that this was a common practice in Britain.[27] However, the consultant who was attacked, rightly argued that it was illogical to ask for consent and to proceed to give ECT, notwithstanding a refusal, as recommended in the memorandum.[28]

The use of ECT by force is constantly being justified by psychiatrists on "humanistic" grounds. This itself is an indication of dehumanisation. Those who disagree with them tend to be described as "maverick psychiatrists" who do not see that "a patient's refusal or inability to consent to treatment is itself a symptom of his disease."[29] One of the advocates of compulsory ECT expressed it in the following circular argument: "If necessary, I should want ECT given against my will." Salzman was correct in suggesting that ultimately civil libertarians and the public must be included in discussions attempting to set ethical guidelines for the use of ECT.[30]

The practice of ECT administration in Great Britain was described as "deeply disturbing" by a Lancet editorialist.[31] Attendant staff is generally hostile to ECT[27] and view the procedure as controlling and punishing the patients.[24] The report on the abuses of ECT in the St. Augustine Hospital in Canterbury contains accounts such as: "a patient in a depressed state was refusing to have ECT ... three nurses went to fetch him and half-dragged half-carried him ... struggling and pleading."[32]

Nine signatories accused the media of falsely presenting ECT by "some ancient film of straight ECT from the days of Cerietti and Bini."[33] They admitted implicitly that not all was fair in the old days. A few years ago a scandal erupted in Britain after the discovery that unmodified ECT was used in Broadmoor Hospital to "control" patients' behaviour. This was defended by the President of the Royal College of Psychiatrists and by others.[34,35] The Lancet commented that "the cuckoo's nest may not be as empty as we supposed."[34]

For most patients the threat of being put on the shock list has the instant effect of bringing their conduct into line.[36] In a Vietnamese hospital under U.S. control, the whole ward of male patients were given the option to work or to get straight ECT. It was not clear how many ultimately opted for work because of the fear of ECT, but the "mass treatment" worked. In the female ward, shocking patients into work did not achieve its objective, despite 20 shocks per person, but starving them for 3 days was successful. Dr. Cotter, who carried out these "behavioural modifications" expressed the opinion that "inflicting a little discomfort was well justified."[37] Since this type of report appears in the official psychiatric journals, one may be forgiven for doubts whether psychiatrists alone are able to maintain self-discipline among their ranks.

In Britain, black mental patients are more likely to receive ECT than the whites.[38] Again and again, the use of ECT as a means of controlling behaviour, against the wishes of the patient and the family, is advocated.[39] With the instrument at hand, a button inviting to be pressed, and the unlimited power to use it, the moral corruption of its users is inevitable. Most scandals of ECT abuse are brought to light not by psychiatrists involved or their colleagues, but by auxiliary staff, or the patients themselves. "It is not ECT which has brought psychiatry into disrepute. Psychiatry has done just that for ECT."[31]

In the past, psychiatrists did not draw a sharp line between treatment and punishment. Cameron of the Midlothian District Asylum in Edinburgh used hyoscyamine to teach patients good behaviour. "The patient lies in a state of profound coma, with swollen livid features, widely dilated pupils, and slow, stertorous, almost convulsive breathing... One remarkable feature in the effects produced by hyoscyamine... is the extreme repugnance with which it is regarded by all who have experienced its effects... it is of wonderful efficacy in some cases of persistent mischievous behaviour."[40]

Empiricism of convulsive treatment

Sakel, Meduna, and Cerletti, the fathers of modern shock therapy, were no scientists. Their writings are characterised by muddled thinking, bizarre theorising, and egocentric striving for fame. They discovered no new principles of treatment and no new understanding of psychoses. The common denominator of their therapeutic efforts was the ancient notion of shocking patients back to sanity. There is a streak of cruelty in their use of patients to advance their own fame. It was the Zeitgeist of the late thirties (so accurately captured by Karl Kraus in *Die Dritte Walpurgisnacht* in 1933) which allowed and applauded the revival of shock therapy in mental asylums. It is hardly a coincidence that the convulsive therapies and psychosurgery all emerged and gained a wide acceptance in the years 1935-1938.

Sakel from Vienna was the most naive of the three. Using insulin as a sedative in the treatment of neurotics and morphinists, he observed that accidental overdosage of insulin resulted in epileptic fits or coma. Those who survived were "psychically improved." "I began with addicts ... I observed improvements after severe epileptic shocks ... Those patients who had previously been excited and irritable, suddenly become contented and quiet after these shocks... The success I had achieved in treating addicts and neurotics... encouraged me to use it in the treatment of schizophrenia or major psychoses."[41] In 1938, Sakel felt that insulin coma ("wet shock") could be improved by chemically-induced seizures ("dry shock"), since spontaneous convulsions after insulin were unpredictable. He experimented with strychnine, camphor and cardiazol. As he saw it, "the epileptic fit is the artillery, the hypoglycaemia is the infantry in the battle against the disease."[42,43] Joseph Wortis, who acted as Sakel's interpreter, recorded that, according to one critical observer, Sakel "spun some really fancy theories ... naive mixture of physics, chemistry, physiology, and circumlocution."[44]

Meduna, experimenting independently on patients in a Hungarian state mental asylum, was influenced by his chief, Professor Nyirö, who previously tried (unsuccessfully) to cure schizophrenia by injections of blood from epileptics. The first of Meduna's experiments (camphor-induced shocks) were a repetition of the 16th century treatment for lunacy by Paracelsus. Meduna attacked Sakel's method as lacking a sound theoretical basis.[45] For a short period, Meduna defended the use of chemical-induced epileptic convulsions by an antagonism between schizophrenia and epilepsy. He believed that the equilibrium between mesoderm and ectoderm was disturbed both in epilepsy and schizophrenia, but in opposite directions.[45] This nonsensical theory was abandoned by Meduna one year later, when he finally admitted that it is the "shock" which matters. He suggested that his method is like "water-shock" therapy in uraemia in that shocking the brain of a schizophrenic stimulates "a sluggishly reacting organ to maximum effort."[46] While Sakel thought in terms of bombardment of the brain,

Meduna spoke of "dynamite, endeavouring to blow asunder the pathological sequences... We are undertaking a violent onslaught...because at present nothing less than such a shock to the organism is powerful enough to break the chain of noxious processes that leads to schizophrenia."[45]

Others thought that the main effect of convulsive therapy was "to knock out, transiently or permanently, diseased nerve-cells which are less resistant than healthy cells."[12] The vocabulary has been borrowed from cancer treatment. Mental disease was a cancer of the mind, or rather, of the brain.

Cerletti discovered nothing, since he started to use electrically-induced fits only after epileptic treatment of schizophrenia had been promoted by Sakel and Meduna. Cerletti himself stated that "except for the fortuitous and fortunate circumstances of pigs' pseudo-butchery, electro-shock would not have been born."[21] This is not accurate, since at his time there was an extensive literature on induction of epilepsy by electric current (reviewed for example by Ward and Clark[47]).

Galvani's nephew, Aldini, was reported to have cured two cases of melancholia by passing galvanic current through the brain in 1804.[48] In England, Clifford Allbutt in 1872 used the passage of electric current through the head for treatment of mania, brain-wasting, dementia and melancholia.[49] In 1876, Savage recorded that melancholia improved after an epileptic fit. In 1885, de Watteville wrote that "the application of electricity to the treatment of insanity is, I am happy to observe, beginning to occupy the attention of alienist."[50] The first experiments in inducing epileptic fits by direct needling of the brain with an electrode (in an Irish immigrant to the USA) were carried out by Bartholow in 1874.[51] The history of the use of electricity in treatment of insanity is reviewed by Harms[52] and Mowbray.[53] Löwenfeld achieved induction of epileptic fits by passing electric current through the head of his mental patients.[54] The idea was old and primitive. "It is said that the Abyssinians make use of the torpedo for the cure of fevers. They tie the patient on his back on a table and apply the fish to all parts of the body. The operation is attended with extreme torture, but they pretend that it carries off the disease." as recorded in 1796.[55]

The bizarre experimentation of Cerletti can be illustrated by his "discovery" that mental patients improve remarkably after injection of brain matter from animals treated with electroshock. Cerletti advocated the method of "annihilation" introduced by his colleague, Bini, in 1942, which consisted in giving a series of ECT many times a day for many days.[21] This reduced the patient to a vegetable state. Patients became incontinent and they required artificial feeding. Cerletti observed that the annihilation method gave "good" results in obsessive states, in psychogenic depression, and even in paranoid states.[21] Ten years ago this method, under a euphemism of "regressive ECT," was still advocated by some American psychiatrists.[56]

Cerletti believed that he had discovered a panacea: he reported ECT as successful in toxicomania, progressive paralysis, Parkinsonism, disseminated sclerosis, asthma, psoriasis, itch, oezena and alopecia.[21] His followers used ECT to "cure" homosexuals.[12] As pointed out by Cook,[12] there was more than a touch of irony in the fact that convulsion treatment, introduced as a specific measure against schizophrenia was found to be specific for affective psychoses. ECT is still used in anorexia nervosa, obsessional illnesses, organic confusional states, and psychogenic pain, without any rationale.[57] A recent survey of the usage of ECT in Massachusetts found that in 1980 in general hospitals, 42% of ECT administrations were in "dysthymic disorder" (which includes depressive neurosis) and only 16% for major depression.[58] Mills et al. thought that at least 20% of patients received ECT for inappropriate indications.[58] It is quite clear from the current psychiatric literature that there is no agreement on what are the appropriate indications. This is not surprising considering the empirical nature of the treatment lacking any explanation why it should work.

Does ECT cause brain damage?

This contentious issue is confounded by several misunderstandings. Firstly, the notion of brain damage was not introduced by the critics of convulsive therapy but by its advocates. Secondly, there is no dispute about ECT causing an acute brain syndrome — the question is whether this "damage" has permanent consequences, and if so, how often and to what degree? Thirdly, no one disputes that ECT impairs memory, but again, the question is one of the type, severity, and duration.

Templer compared appropriately this issue with the debate about the effect of boxing on the brain: "ECT is not the only domain in which damage to the human brain is denied or deemphasised on the grounds that this damage is minor, occurs in a very small percentage of cases, or is primarily a matter of the past."[59] In fact, nearly half of the U.S. psychiatrists believe that ECT produces slight or subtle brain damage.[60]

That insulin coma or metrazol shock can cause brain damage was realised early in the history of convulsive treatment and in the discussion to Weil's paper, Dr. Roy Grinker asked in 1938: "Does shock therapy improve schizophrenic patients by structural damage of a less intense but more diffuse type?"[61] Whether there was a therapeutic value in a certain amount of brain damage was a moot point.[62] Bini at the Münsingen Congress in 1938 reported that the brain damage in experimental animals treated with electroshock was severe and widespread. "The importance of the alterations we have met so far in our animals does not permit us to exclude the possibility of applying these physical methods in human therapy... These very alterations may be responsible for the favourable transformation of the morbid psychic picture of schizophrenia."[63]

The most venomous criticism of convulsive therapy came from Breggin[64] and Friedberg,[65] whose evidence was based mainly on the old literature. Unfortunately, the neuropathological literature is a "morass of poorly done and largely uninterpretable studies."[66] In a superb review of this morass, Weiner found little evidence for permanent brain "damage" but he concluded that memory deficits after ECT do occur and some of them could be persistent.[67] Another abnormality which takes weeks to months to disappear and may persist even longer in rare cases is EEG slowing.[68] The significance of this is not clear. More recently, Calloway and Dolan raised the question of frontal lobe atrophy in patients previously treated with ECT.[69]

Cook in an early exhaustive review of convulsive therapy discussed the post-ECT amnestic syndrome, which varied from "mild forgetfulness to severe confusion of the Korsakow's type" occasionally persisting for long periods.[12] One of the first studies attempting to quantify memory disturbance after convulsive therapy was by Tooth and Blackbourn.[70] However, research methodologies for assessing memory deficits following ECT have been generally inadequate.[71] Kendell in his valuable review found the studies by Janis, Squire, and Freeman as fairly convincing that past memory can be permanently disrupted by ECT.[57] Squire studied patients treated with ECT for depression (i.e., given shorter courses than schizophrenics) and found that information acquired in the days and weeks prior to and just after ECT may be permanently lost. There may be patchy and permanent gaps for events in the 1-2 years preceding ECT. The disruption of recall for events that occurred many years previously recovered virtually completely within 7 months of ECT treatment.[72,73]

In a questionnaire administered to patients who had ECT, 28-30% claimed that their memory never returned to normal and that ECT caused permanent changes to memory.[18] It is possible that gaps in autobiographic memory may have therapeutic value. "Can'st thou not minister to a mind diseased; pluck from the memory a rooted sorrow, raze out the written troubles of the brain" (*Macbeth*, v, iii). In this sense, such memory loss could indeed be welcomed and denoted as "trivial."[74]

There is, however, a strong resistance by the advocates of ECT to accept any criticism, even when it is so meticulously fair as Weiner's. Fink accused Weiner that he "genuflects to avoid criticism" and that "such kowtowing is inappropriate."[74] These intemperate words were seconded by Kalinowsky, who brushed away the criticism with "no need to investigate reasons for a few dissenting voices"[75] The same Kalinowsky dismissed spinal compression fractures occurring during the acute anterior flexion in metrazol shocks in 40-50% of patients[76] as having "no clinical significance."[12]

Fink argues that the principal risks of ECT (amnesia and organic brain syndrome) can be reduced by hyperoxygenation, unilateral placement of the electrodes over the nondominant hemisphere, and use of minimal induction currents.[77] Surely if amnesia and organic brain syndrome were trivial, there should be no reason for these elaborate modifications. Moreover, these very modifications may be responsible for decreasing the efficacy of ECT as noted in several recent trials and studies.

For example, Robin and de Tissera questioned the belief that what matters is the convulsion and not the electric energy required to elicit it.[78] Experiments with unilateral placement of the electrodes started early in attempt to reduce confusion and memory disturbance,[79] but despite the repeated assurance of the equipotency of bilateral and unilateral ECT,[80,81] most psychiatrists have not yet been convinced.[82-84] It is of interest that in Massachusetts in 1980, 90% of ECT in public hospitals were bilateral, though only 39% were bilateral in private hospitals.[58]

Efficacy of ECT

Schizophrenia

Defending ECT against public criticism, the secretary of the Society of Clinical Psychiatrists stated that "sensible people must surely realise that well-trained professionals are not going to continue administering a treatment for many years if it does not work".[85] In the case of schizophrenia, the well-trained professionals have been doing just that for the last 50 years. Kalinowsky still believes that insulin shocks are the best treatment for schizophrenia; his opinion is based on his experience and he dismisses controlled studies as irrelevant.[86] Fink believes that ECT is at least equal to other therapies in schizophrenia, and in support of his claim he quotes obsolete and subjective impressions by Kalinowsky, and Sargant and Slater.[1] In fact, Sargant advocated insulin coma for schizophrenia as late as 1958.[87]

There is no evidence that ECT alters the schizophrenic process.[88] Even the initial enthusiasm for convulsive and insulin treatments in schizophrenia was not universally shared. In 1939, Stalker found no difference in outcome of schizophrenia, regardless of whether insulin shocks, cardiazol shocks, or psychotherapy were used.[89] Meduna's compatriots found cardiazol shocks and insulin shocks worse than no treatment.[90] Bourne brought attention to the fact that schizophrenics treated with insulin received 50-100 times more attention by the staff than the patients not so treated.[91] In the first mammoth review of somatic therapies, using confidence intervals, Appel et al. found that ECT was no better than hospitalisation alone.[92] David found only two controlled studies on the efficacy of insulin treatment: none showed insulin better than placebo.[93] Ackner et al. found no difference between insulin coma and barbiturate sleep.[94] Leyton showed that placebo (i.v. glucose) was as effective as a course of 40 insulin comas.[95] Brill et al. found ECT no better than anaesthesia alone.[16] Riddell, reviewing the literature at the beginning of the sixties, concluded that the era of shock therapy was fast drawing to a close.[96] The only controlled study from recent times on the efficacy of ECT in schizophrenia was carried out by Taylor and Fleminger.[97] Despite their conclusion that ECT was effective in paranoid schizophrenia, no difference was demonstrable 2 months after a short course of treatment. No further improvement was observed after the initial six ECTs, which runs against the clinical lore that on average 20 ECTs are necessary in schizophrenia. The nurses and the relatives could not distinguish between the treated and the control group. These were very unimpressive findings and it is not surprising that 60% of the US psychiatrists consider ECT in schizophrenia as inappropriate.[60] What is more worrying is the source of conviction of the remaining 40% who believe that ECT in schizophrenia is not inappropriate.

Depression

The most often quoted studies demonstrating the effectiveness of ECT in depression have been Greenblatt at al.[98] and the British Medical Research Council study.[99] One wonders how many psychiatrists read more than the abstracts of these studies. Greenblatt et al. reported that ECT was universally effective in depression, regardless of the type: 70-80% of depressed patients improved, including manic-depressives, psychoneurotics, involutional depression, and character disorders. "There were no significant differences among any of the diagnostic groups" treated by ECT, which included also schizoaffective reactions. Placebo response at least equalled imipramine, phenelzine, and isocarboxazid. Greenblatt's study was pooled from 3 hospitals: in hospitals A and C, ECT was as good as imipramine; in hospitals B and C, ECT equalled placebo. The placebo response (markedly or moderately improved) after 8 weeks was 69%. Improvements as high as 70-80% can be expected due to placebo alone.[100]

In the MRC study,[99] at the end of 5 weeks, more male patients were discharged who received placebo than those treated with ECT. No difference was observed in male patients among the four treatment groups (ECT, phenelzine, imipramine, placebo).

In the last seven years seven controlled trials were carried out in Britain. The initial impetus was the memorandum of the Royal College of Psychiatrists[25] issued in response to another report of ECT abuse. The memorandum minimised the side effects of ECT and wishfully declared the evidence for ECT effectiveness in depressive illness as "incontrovertible", though it was admitted that "in depressed patients there is suggestive, if not yet unequivocal evidence that the convulsion is a necessary element in the therapeutic effect."[25] It was this uncertainty which the seven trials tried to resolve, using randomisation of patients to simulated and real ECT. Each trial which threw doubts on the "incontrovertibility" of the evidence was severely attacked by correspondents questioning methodology and even motives of the trialists. There were few questions asked about the methodology (usually much more spurious) of trials more favourable to ECT. One of the commentators was of the opinion that "despite all precautions, the preconceptions of the [trialists] somehow influenced their findings."[57]

Freeman et al.[101] went only one third of the way: only the first two ECTs of six were simulated in the control group. Treatment was discontinued for reasons other than satisfactory response in six of 20 in the real ECT group and in only two of 20 in the sham ECT group. The trial was unsatisfactory. Lambourn and Gill[102] used unilateral ECT (simulated and real) — they found no difference. The Northwick Park trial,[103] considered by many as the best trial yet, showed no difference between the simulated and real ECT at one and six-month follow-up. After a four-week treatment period, the advantage of real ECT showed in only one of three rating scales used. The authors suggested that good nursing care and medical care can be equally good. This was counteracted by West,[104] who found real ECT superior to simulated ECT. It was not stated how the single author carried out the double-blinding procedure. The uncertainty was strengthened by the lack of any improvement in the control group during the three-week treatment period. Gangadhar et al.[105] compared ECT (and placebo) with simulated ECT (and imipramine): both treatments produced equally significant improvements which were maintained for the duration of 6-month follow-up. Brandon et al.[106] confirmed the findings of the Northwick Park trial. Both simulated and real ECT resulted in significant improvements. At the end of four-week treatment, consultants were unable to guess who received real or simulated ECT. The initial difference in favour of real ECT disappeared at 12 and 28 weeks. In the latest trial, Gregory et al.[107] compared simulated ECT with unilateral and bilateral ECT. After a two-week treatment period, bilateral and unilateral ECT groups improved faster than the simulated-ECT group, but there was no difference one, three, and six months after the trial. This trial is more difficult to evaluate since all groups received additional ECT after the end of the trial. The trial was marred by a high rate of drop-outs: only 64% patients completed the study and an equal number withdrew from the simulated and bilateral ECT groups.

In his thoughtful review, Crow questioned the widely held view that the convulsion is a necessary component of the therapeutic effect of ECT.[108] He also raised the important question whether there are certain types of depression which respond to ECT only. From the material of the Northwick Park trial,[103] it appears that only depressed patients with delusions responded more to real ECT than to simulated ECT.[104] This would narrow the indications for ECT a great deal. There was no evidence that endogenous features were sufficient predictors of response to ECT. These findings are important and should be replicated. It is, however, doubtful, whether in delusional depression, ECT should be the treatment of choice. Spiker et al. showed that in delusional depression the combination of amitriptyline and perphenazine is probably at least as good as ECT.[110]

The question then remains, is ECT necessary as a treatment modality in psychiatry? From the earliest times of convulsive therapy, it was recognised that the treatment is unspecific and consists in shortening the duration of the illness rather than in improving the outcome.[111] One of the arguments for retaining ECT is the prevention of suicides in depressed patients. The standard reference given to support this view is the paper by Avery and Winokur.[112] Close reading of this report reveals that the patients who received ECT and antidepressants had a suicide rate twice that of patients who received antidepressants only. Moreover, the study shows that there was no difference between the suicide rate in patients treated with either ECT or with antidepressants. More recently, Babigian and Guttmacher[113] found that the duration of hospitalisation of depressed patients who received ECT was on average about twice that of those who did not receive ECT. The mortality risk for suicide was the same for both groups. ECT recipients died sooner after the first hospitalisation than patients who did not receive ECT. While these results are difficult to interpret because of the problem of selection, they do not lend support for the notion that ECT prevents suicides. Similarly, Fernando and Storm[114] found no significant difference in the rate of suicide between patients who received ECT and those who did not. Thus, the suicide argument does not stand up.

Conclusions

Convulsive therapy is a primitive and unspecific treatment, initially based on the old belief of shocking the patient into sanity.

Recent controlled trials suggest that ECT shortens the duration of recovery in depressive illness, particularly in the delusional variety, but it is clear that the large proportion of the improvement attributed to ECT is a placebo effect or possibly the effect of anaesthesia. Undoubtedly, electrically or chemically induced seizures have a profound, but short-lived, effect on brain function (acute organic brain syndrome), which affects performance in the rating tests by which mental disease is quantified. There is, however, no evidence that these functional and biochemical changes affect specifically and fundamentally the underlying psychopathology of psychoses.

It is difficult not to accept the general consensus that ECT is a relatively safe procedure with little long-term effect. While ECT has not been shown to be superior to drugs, it must be taken into account that the side-effects of drugs are not negligible, and are often more serious than those of ECT. However, because of strong pressures from some psychiatrists to use ECT against the will of the patient or his relatives, the temptation to use ECT indiscriminately, and the inevitable abuse of ECT as a means of punishment by a small minority of irresponsible psychiatrists who wield the power to do so, the use of ECT should be restricted by law and controlled by selected bodies representing both the public and the psychiatric profession.

References

1. Fink M. Myths of "shock therapy". *Am J Psychiat* 1977; 134: 991-6.
2. Ackerknecht EH. A short history of psychiatry. 2nd ed. Hafner, New York, 1968: 102.
3. Pascal C, Davesne J. Traitement des maladies mentales par les chocs. Masson, Paris, 1926: 182.
4. Menzies D. Pyrotherapy in dementia praecox. *Lancet* 1935; ii: 994-6.
5. Sargant W, Slater E. An introduction to physical methods of treatment in psychiatry. Livingstone, Edinburgh, 1944: 52.
6. Rather LJ. Mind and body in eighteenth century medicine. Wellcome Historical Medical Library, London, 1965: 187.
7. Savage GH. Cases of insanity relieved by acute disease. *Practitioner* 1876; 16: 449-53.

8   Winslow F. On the medical treatment of insanity.
     J Psychol Med Ment Sci 1854; 7: 205-39.
9   Skultans V. Madness and morals. Ideas on insanity in the 19th century.
     Routledge & Kegan Paul, London, 1975: 120-46.
10   Winslow F. Prolonged shower-baths in the treatment of the insane.
     J Psychol Med Ment Sci 1857; 10: 1-28.
11   Meduna L, Friedman E. The convulsive-irritative therapy of the psychoses. *JAMA* 1939; 112: 501-9.
12   Cook LC. Convulsion therapy. *J Ment Sci* 1944; 90: 435-64.
13   Low AA, Sonenthal LR, Blaurock MF, Kaplan M, Sherman I. Metrazol shock treatment of the "functional" psychoses.
     Arch Neurol Psychiat 1938; 39: 717-35.
14   Cook LC. Cardiazol convulsion therapy in schizophrenia.
     Proc Roy Soc Med 1938; 31: 567-77.
15   Humbert F, Friedemann A. Critique and indications of treatments in schizophrenia. *Am J Psychiat* 1938; 94 suppl: 176-83.
16   Brill HQ, Crumpton E, Eiduson S, Grayston HM, Hellman LI, Richards RA. Relative effectiveness of various components of electroconvulsive therapy. *Arch Neuro Psychiat* 1959; 81: 627-35.
17   Hobson JA., Prescott F. Use of d-tubocurarine chloride and thiopentone in electroconvulsive therapy. *Br Med J* 1947; i: 445-8.
18   Freeman CPL, Kendell RE. ECT.I. Patients' experiences and attitudes.
     Br J Psychiat 1980; 137: 8-16.
19   Fink M. Antipsychiatrists and ECT. *Br Med J* 1976; i: 280.
20   Impastato DJ. The story of the first electroshock treatment.
     Am J Psychiat 1959; 116: 1113-4.
21   Cerletti U. Old and new information about electroshock.
     Am J Psychiat 1950; 107: 87-94.
22   Fink M. Meduna and the origins of convulsive therapy.
     Am J Psychiat 1984; 141:1034-41.
23   Greenblatt M. Efficacy of ECT in affective and schizophrenic illness.
     Am J Psychiat 1977; 134: 1001-5.
24   Levenson JL, Willett AB. Milieu reactions to ECT.
     Psychiatry 1982; 45: 298-306.
25   Anonymous. The Royal College of Psychiatrists' Memorandum on the

use of electroconvulsive therapy. *Br J Psychiat* 1977; 131: 261-72.

26 Anonymous. College memorandum on ECT (editorial comment). *Br J Psychiat* 1977; 131: 647-8.

27 Pippard J. Ellam L. Electroconvulsive treatment in Great Britain. *Br J Psychiat* 1981; 139: 563-8.

28 Spencer S. College memorandum on ECT. *Br J Psychiat* 1977; 131: 645-6.

29 Lynch T. Electroconvulsive therapy. *Ir Med J* 1981; 74: 29.

30 Salzman C. ECT and ethical psychiatry. *Am J Psychiat* 1977; 134: 1006-9.

31 Anonymous. ECT in Britain: a shameful state of affairs. *Lancet* 1981; ii: 1207-8.

32 Watt DC. Compulsory electroconvulsive therapy. *Lancet* 1976; ii: 736.

33 Anderson JF, Sethi P, MacDonald EJ, et al. ECT and the media. *Br Med J* 1977; 2: 1081-2.

34 Anonymous. ECT in Broadmoor. *Lancet* 1980; i: 348-9.

35 Crammer J. Unmodified ECT. *Lancet* 1980; i: 486.

36 Belknap I. Human problems in a state mental hospital. New York: McGraw-Hill, 1956; 191-4.

37 Cotter LH. Operant conditioning in a Vietnamese mental hospital. *Am J Psychiat* 1967; 124: 23-8.

38 Anonymous. Black and white health. *Lancet* 1984; ii: 115.

39 Jeffries JJ, Rakoff VM. ECT as a form of restraint. *Can J Psychiat* 1983; 28: 661-3.

40 Cameron WD. The philosophy of restraint in the management of the insane. *J Ment Sci* 1883; 28: 519-31.

41 Sakel M. Schizophrenia. Owen, London, 1959: 188-228.

42 Sakel M. The nature and origin of the hypoglycemic treatment of psychoses. *Am J Psychiat* 1938; 94 suppl: 24-40.

43 Sakel M. Historique de l'origine du traitement de la schizophrénie par le choc insulinique. *L'Encéphale* 1938; 33: 153-54.

44 Wortis J. How shock treatment came to America: What history teaches. *Biol Psychiat* 1982; 17: 1203-4.

45 Meduna L. General discussion of the cardiazol therapy. *Am J Psychiat* 1938; 94 suppl: 40-50.

46 Meduna L, Rohny B. Insulin and cardiazol treatment of schizophrenia. *Lancet* 1939; i: 1039-42.

47 Ward JW, Clark SL. Convulsions produced by electrical stimulation of the cerebral cortex. *Arch Neurol Psychiat* 1938; 39: 1213-27.

48 Newth AH. The value of electricity on the treatment of insanity. *J Ment Sci* 1885; 30: 354-9.

49 Anonymous. A review of Browne JC (ed): The West Riding Lunatic Asylum Medical Report, 1872. *Practitioner* 1872; 9: 362-4.

50 de Watteville A. Practical remarks on the use of electricity in mental disease. *J Ment Sci* 1895; 30: 483-8.

51 Morgan JP. The first reported case of electrical stimulation of the human brain. *J Hist Med* 1982; 37: 51-64.

52 Harms E. The origin and early history of electrotherapy and electroshock. *Am J Psychiat* 1955; 111: 933.4.

53 Mowbray RM. Historical aspects of electric convulsant therapy. *Scot Med J* 1959; 4: 373-8.

54 Anonymous. A review of two books by L. Löwenfeld. *J Ment Sci* 1884; 39: 415-24.

55 "A letter from M. Iberti to one of his friends". *Med Chirurg Rev* 1796; 2: 18-24.

56 Exner J, Murillo L. Effectiveness of regressive ECT with process schizophrenia. *Dis Nerv Syst* 1973; 34: 44-8.

57 Kendell RE. The present status of electroconvulsive therapy. *Br J Psychiat* 1981; 139: 265-83.

58 Mills MJ, Pearsall DT, Yesavage JA, Salzman C. Electroconvulsive therapy in Massachusetts. *Am J Psychiat* 1984; 141: 534-8.

59 Templer DI. ECT and brain damage: How much risk is acceptable? *Behav Brain Sci* 1984; 7: 39.

60 American Psychiatric Association. Task Force on Electroconvulsive Therapy. Report 14. Washington. 1978.

61 Weil A, Liebert E, Heilbrunn G. Histopathological changes in the brain in experimental hyperinsulinism. *Arch Neurol Psychiat* 1938; 39: 467-81.

62 Tennent T. Insulin therapy. *J Ment Sci* 1944: 90: 465-85.

63 Bini L. Experimental researches in epileptic attacks induced by electric

current. *Am J Psychiat* 1938; 94 suppl: 172-3.

64 Breggin PR. Disabling the brain with electroshock. In: Doniger M, Wittkower ED, eds. Divergent views in psychiatry. Harper & Row, Hagerstown, 1981: 247-71.

65 Friedberg J. Shock treatment, brain damage, and memory loss: a neurological perspective. *Am J Psychiat* 1977; 134: 1010-4.

66 Weiner RD. The psychiatric use of electrically induced seizures. *Am J Psychiat* 1979; 136: 1507-17.

67 Weiner RD. Does electroconvulsive therapy cause brain damage? (A target article with 22 commentaries.) *Behav Brain Sci* 1984; 7: 1-54.

68 Weiner RD. The persistence of electroconvulsive therapy-induced changes in the electroencephalogram. *J Nerv Ment Dis* 1980; 168: 224-8.

69 Calloway SP, Dolan R. ECT and cerebral damage. *Br J Psychiat* 1982; 140: 103.

70 Tooth G, Blackbourn JM. Disturbance of memory after convulsion treatment. *Lancet* 1939; ii: 17-20.

71 Harper RG, Wiens AN. Electroconvulsive therapy and memory. *J Nerv Ment Dis* 1975; 161: 245-54.

72 Squire LR, Slater PC, Miller PL. Retrograde amnesia and bilateral electroconvulsive therapy. *Arch Gen Psychiat* 1981; 38: 89-95.

73 Squire LR. Opinions and facts about ECT: Can science help? *Behav Brain Sci* 1984: 7: 34-7.

74 Fink M. ECT - verdict: not guilty. *Behav Brain Sci* 1984; 7: 26-7.

75 Kalinowsky LB. Problems in research on electroconvulsive therapy. *Behav Brain Sci* 1984; 7: 28-9.

76 Polatin P, Friedman MM, Harris MM, Horwitz WA. Vertebral fractures produced by metrazol-induced convulsions. *JAMA* 1939; 112: 1684-7.

77 Fink M. Convulsive and drug therapies of depression. *Ann Rev Med* 1981; 32: 405-12.

78 Robin A, de Tissera S. A double-blind controlled comparison of the therapeutical effects of low and high energy electroconvulsive therapies. *Br J Psychiat* 1982, 141: 357-66.

79 Pacella BL, Impastato DJ. Focal stimulation therapy. *Am J Psychiat* 1954; 116: 576-8.

80   d'Elia G, Raothma H. Is unilateral ECT less effective than bilateral ECT? *Br J Psychiat* 1975; 126: 83-9.

81   Fontaine R, Young T. Unilateral ECT: advantages and efficacy in the treatment of depression. *Can J Psychiat* 1985; 30: 142-7.

82   Abrams R, Taylor MA. Diencephalic stimulation and the effects of ECT in endogenous depression. *Br J Psychiat* 1976; 129: 482-5.

83   Kalinowsky LB. Simulated and real ECT. *Br J Psychiat* 1979; 134:647-52.

84   Sackeim HA. Not all seizures are created equal: the importance of ECT dose-response variables. *Behav Brain Sci* 1984; 7: 32-3.

85   Haslam MT. ECT on television. *Br Med J* 1977; 2: 455.

86   Kalinowsky LB. Biological psychiatric treatment preceding pharmacotherapy. In: Ayd FJ, Blackwell B. eds. Discoveries in biological psychiatry. Lippincott, Philadelphia, 1970: 59-67.

87   Sargant W. Insulin coma for schizophrenia. *Lancet* 1958; ii: 1370-1.

88   Salzman C. The use of ECT in the treatment of schizophrenia. *Am J Psychiat* 1980; 137: 1032-41.

89   Stalker H, Millar WM. Jacobs JM. Remissions in schizophrenia. Insulin and convulsion therapies compared with ordinary treatment. *Lancet* 1939; i: 437-9.

90   Lehoczky, Horányi, Eszenyi, Bak. Disturbance of memory after convulsion treatment. *Lancet* 1939; ii: 283.

91   Bourne H. The insulin myth. *Lancet* 1953; ii: 964-8.

92   Appel KE, Myers MJ, Scheflen AE. Prognosis in psychiatry: results of psychiatric treatment. *Arch Neurol Psychiat* 1953; 70: 459-68.

93   David HP. A critique of psychiatric and psychological research on insulin treatment in schizophrenia. *Am J Psychiat* 1954; 110: 774-5.

94   Ackner B, Harris A, Oldham AJ. Insulin treatment of schizophrenia. A controlled study. *Lancet* 1957; i: 607-11.

95   Leyton SR. Glucose and insulin in schizophrenia. *Lancet* 1958; i: 1253-4.

96   Riddell SA. The therapeutic efficacy of ECT. *Arch Gen Psychiat* 1963; 8: 548-.56.

97   Taylor P, Fleminger JJ. ECT for schizophrenia. *Lancet* 1980; i: 1380-3.

98   Greenblatt M, Grosser GH, Wechsler H. Differential response of hospitalized depressed patients to somatic therapy. *Am J Psychiat* 1964; 120: 935-43.

99   Medical Research Council Psychiatric Committee. Clinical trial of the treatment of depressive illness. *Br Med J* 1965; i: 881-6.

100 Lowinger P, Dobie S. A study of placebo response rates. *Arch Gen Psychiat* 1969; 20: 84-8.

101 Freeman CPL, Basson JV, Crighton A. Double-blind controlled trial of electroconvulsive therapy (ECT) and simulated ECT in depressive illness. *Lancet* 1978; i: 738-40.

102 Lambourn J, Gill D. A controlled comparison of simulated and real ECT. *Br J Psychiat* 1978; 133: 514-9.

103 Johnstone EC, Deakin JFW, Lawler P, Frith CD, Stevens M, McPherson K, Crow TJ. The Northwick Park electroconvulsive therapy trial. *Lancet* 1980; ii: 1317-20.

104 West ED. Electric stimulation therapy in depression: a double-blind controlled trial. *Br Med J* 1981; 282: 355-7.

105 Gangadhar BN, Kapur RL, Kalyanasundaram S. Comparison of electroconvulsive therapy with imipramine in endogenous depression: a double-blind study. *Br J Psychiat* 1982; 141: 367-71.

106 Brandon S, Cowley P, MaDonald C, Neville P, Palmer R, Wellstood-Eason S. Electroconvulsive therapy; results in depressive illness from the Leicestershire trial. *Br Med J* 1984; 288: 22-5.

107 Gregory S, Shawcross CR, Gill D. The Nottingham ECT study. A double-blind comparison of bilateral, unilateral, and simulated ECT in depressive illness *Br J Psychiat* 1985; 146; 520-4.

108 Crow TJ. The scientific status of electro-convulsive therapy. *Psychol Med* 1979; 9: 401-8.

109 Crow TJ, Deakin JFW, Johnstone EC. The Northwick Park ECT trial. Predictors of response to real and simulated ECT. *Br J Psychiat* 1984; 144: 227-37.

110 Spiker DG, Weiss JC, Dealy RS, Griffin SJ, Hanin I, Neil JF, Perel JM, Rossi AJ, Soloff PH. The pharmacological treatment of delusional depression. *Am J Psychiat* 1985. 142: 430-1.

111 Anonymous. Convulsion therapy. (Editorial) *Lancet* 1939; 1: 457.

112 Avery D, Winokur G. Mortality in depressed patients treated with electroconvulsive therapy and antidepressants. *Arch Gen Psychiat* 1976; 33: 1029-37.

113 Babigian HM, Guttmacher LB. Epidemiological considerations in electroconvulsive therapy. *Arch Gen Psychiat* 1984; 41: 246-53.

114 Fernando S, Storm V. Suicide among psychiatric patients of a district general hospital. *Psychol Med* 1984; 14: 661-72.

5

FROM LANGUAGE TO LESION

In this essay I wish to explore the consequences of Szasz's seminal idea that the mind cannot be "diseased," except in a metaphorical sense. As with many great intellectual discoveries, the idea is simple, yet it escaped all until spelled out by Szasz. Most psychiatrists still seem unable or unwilling to differentiate among the philosophical, logical, semantic, and pragmatic levels of this idea. In a metaphorical sense, Szasz (the name means "Saxon" derived from "sax," the fearful weapon of the early Saxons), by using his scalpel-sharp language, has inflicted an incurable lesion on the body of psychiatry.

The Brain and the mind

> Doctors will never understand why a brain has incoherent ideas; they will understand no better why another brain has regular and consistent ideas. They will believe themselves to be wise, and they will be as mad as the lunatic. (Voltaire)

In Roger Sperry's analogy, comparing the brain to the TV set and the mind to TV programs, "nothing in electron physics can explain the sequencing of the TV program, that is, the plot developed in a movie, the content of the news, or the comedian's delivery" (Sperry, 1988). The human brain, in distinction to the TV set, generates within itself its mental "programs," whose content cannot be explained by the brain's "software" or "hardware."

Among philosophers of the mind, there is a widespread morbid fear of being labelled Platonic or Cartesian dualists, and thus tainted with the religious and spiritual overtones of such a position. Searle (1992) has had to defend the existence of consciousness and intention (beliefs,

---

This paper was first published in a special issue of the *Review of Existential Psychology and Psychiatry*, Volume XXIII, Nos 1,2,3 (1987)

desires, hopes, fears) against philosophical materialist-reductionists, who maintain that mental events are identical with brain events, thus reducing psychology to neurophysiology. The same reductionism is now the dogma of biological psychiatry. M. Merzenich, of the Institute of Integrated Neurosciences, University of California, San Francisco, stated that "the laws of psychology that govern behaviour are really brain laws ... and the main determinants of these laws are genetic" (Cotton, 1930a).

While the mind cannot be separated from the brain, it does not follow that the mind is an *objective* part of the brain. As Searle put it, while consciousness is real, it is an "ontologically subjective" property of the mind and cannot be defined in psychological terms, exactly because it is a subjective experience.

It is paradoxical that in the past twenty years, while philosophers of the mind have moved away from the reductionist-deterministic notion that the brain controls the mind, toward a more accommodating concept of the mentalist-cognitive model, allowing two-way traffic between mind and brain, and postulating brain "plasticity" (Sperry, 1988), psychiatrists, during the same period, have largely discarded what they thought to be psychological ballast, and have embraced instead brain sciences and genetics.

Biological psychiatry denies that man is a moral agent. However, if mental processes (thoughts, theories, intentions, values, emotions) played no causal role in human behaviour and were only correlates or epiphenomena of brain events, there would be no evolutionary reason for their emergence, since they would lack biological value. This is Popper's view, who advocates the interactionism between brain and mind and warns against the political danger of the utopian dreams of determinists, who believe that all behaviour will be ultimately predictable and explainable by genes and environment (Popper, 1965; 1978).

Since mental processes and behaviour are also studied by psychologists, their reduction to brain events would make psychology redundant. The very existence of psychotherapy, with its implicit evidence that "mental" patients are moral agents, presents an unwelcome competition to biological psychiatrists. Moreover, with psychologists, nonmedical therapists, and psychiatrists working in the same field, it is hard to convince the public that psychiatrists are "real" doctors and scientists. This state of affairs is one of the reasons for the adoption of the medical model by psychiatrists and for their keenness to establish a complex nosological system. However, by abandoning mind and embracing brain, psychiatrists are working toward the abolition of their own discipline. "It is as much nonsense to talk about the physiological causes of meaningful deeds as it is to talk about the mechanics of writing causing the meaning of the poem. The claim of biological psychiatrists that schizophrenia has a physiological cause is as ludicrous as claiming that Nobel Prize-winning literature has a physiological cause" (Leifer, 1982). By claiming that "mental illness is just as any other illness," biological psychiatrists miss the whole point of human behaviour as meaningful activity. If a behaviour is odd, bizarre, crazy, incomprehensible, and so forth, it does not follow that, therefore, it has no meaning or subjective purpose for the person who behaves in such a way. In the medical model, it is meaningless to ask what is the meaning of having multiple sclerosis, since one does not contract a disease because of the need to act out, to act "as if," to rebel, to vent one's frustration, or to respond to the loss of self-esteem and the realization of being a failure. No amount of studies in disciplines as diverse as biochemistry, radiology, endocrinology, neuroanatomy, immunology, pharmacology, or genetics, to name just a few areas with which biological psychiatrists flirt, will throw any light on the meaning and purpose of people's behaviour, however crazy that behaviour may seem to some observers. Similarly, no useful information about the reasons for people becoming depressed, anxious, or addicted to drugs can be gathered from the response to pharmacological treatment. Lack of aspirin is not the cause of fever, lack of water is not the cause of fire. It is irrelevant to the issue in question to argue that some mental disturbances are symptoms of somatic disease.

By playing "scientists," psychiatrists forget that medicine, if they wish to remain within its fold, is not a science but a way of caring for the sick, and also a normalizing discipline, whose norms are determined culturally and ideologically. The difference between a scientist and a psychiatrist is in their approach to reality: one enquires into "what is," while the other is motivated by the question, "What should be done?" The scientist may move from an objective lesion to naming it; while the psychiatrist argues from a subjective description to a lesion, crossing the boundary from mind to brain, and thus committing a categorical error. The psychiatrist also commits what could be called the retrograde naturalist fallacy by arguing from what "ought not to be" (e.g., "mental illness") to "what is" (that is, a hypothetical brain lesion).

What scientific purpose is served by labelling a smoker as suffering from "substance use disorder," specifically, "305.1 tobacco dependence," which can be "continuous, episodic, in remission, or unspecified" (*Diagnostic and Statistical Manual of Mental Disorders III [DSM-III]*)? Would smoking behaviour be better understood by peering into the brain of smokers? Is smoking a disease as any other disease? Could it be that psychiatrists do not see the absurdity of their nosological system?

What is mental disease?

It is useful to distinguish between "disease," as a pathological, somatic process, and "illness," as the subjective feeling of being unwell. Socially unacceptable, aberrant, or "crazy" behaviour does not fit into either of these categories. Many so-called mental patients do not feel "sick," that is, do not have an illness (which, in the jargon of psychiatry is called "lack of insight"), and could not have a disease of the mind, except in a metaphorical sense. Another distinction between "illness" and "disease," in the medical model, is the response to placebo: only illness is modified, leaving the objective lesions (a tubercle, a rheumatoid lesion, a cancer metastasis) unchanged. As psychotherapy is a placebo *par excellence*, and mental patients respond to such therapy, it is further evidence that such patients do not have a "disease."

It serves no purpose to call behaviours, such as wanton destruction of property, arson, rape, and the fear of constrained spaces, diseases or illnesses. A patient with Alzheimer's dementia has a brain disease and may or may not feel ill. When his behaviour transgresses social and legal norms he may need physical restraint or involuntary admission to a hospital, where he is not to be "treated" for a "mental" illness but to be kept in a safe place. His behaviour is exonerated on the basis of mental incompetence. His abnormal behaviour is a *symptom* of the brain disease, just as delirium in a person with high fever or in alcoholic intoxication is a symptom of the underlying serious metabolic disturbance.

The chief difference between medical diagnosis and psychiatric diagnosis is the possibility of objective verification in the former. Thus, for example, "hepatitis E" is an enterally transmitted infection, whose agent has been cloned, and specific tests exist to demonstrate its presence. This is true whether the patient is the President of the United States or a schizophrenic. On the other hand, "undersocialized, nonaggressive conduct disorder," to pick randomly a psychiatric label, has no real meaning. No objective, specific, culture-independent tests exist to verify its presence. The intervals between publishing successive diagnostic manuals of psychiatric diseases ("disorders") are getting shorter, and the number of possible labels is steadily increasing: *DSM-I* (1952) had 106 diagnoses; *DSM-II* (1968), 182; *DSM-III* (1980), 265; *DSM-IIIR* (1987), 292 (Sarbin, 1990). All kinds of nonconforming, undesirable, deviant, incomprehensible, or crazy behaviours are arbitrarily subclassified into hundreds of "disorders," claimed to be "diseases as any other." Whether it is called "disorder" or "disease," behaviour can be described as pathological only in a metaphorical sense; it may be described more accurately as approved or disapproved, moral or immoral, licit or illicit, rational or irrational, since its assessments are determined not by brain neuropathology but by the moral, legal, and societal norms of any given society. Seeing the Virgin Mary on a blank wall and communicating with her is presumably accompanied by the same brain events as seeing and conversing with a Martian. The fact that, in the former case, the phenomenon is interpreted by millions as a miracle, while in the latter case, the interlocutor is likely to receive the label of schizophrenia, makes it clear that it is the meaning attributed to behaviours by other minds which makes the difference, rather than an objective biological event in the mind of the hallucinating person.

To argue, as M. Roth has done (1976), that schizophrenia is a brain disease, just as Parkinsonism was a brain disease even before its neuropathology was elucidated, is disingenuous, since Parkinsonism was not initially understood as a mental disease but a neurological disorder ("shaking palsy"). Charcot's absurd theory, which Roth invokes, that Parkinsonism was caused by political upheaval, does not make the neurological signs of the disease any more "mental."

By assuming that "mental disease" means a not yet discovered brain disease, the biological psychiatrists not only beg the question, but provide the strongest argument against the existence of "mental disease" by implying that it is a *symptom* of brain disease, and therefore not a "disease as any other" but related to a disease, like fever to meningitis or cough to pneumonia. The difference with somatic diseases, however, is that such diseases have other somatic symptoms, while "mental diseases" are symptoms of imaginary brain diseases, which on close inspection disappear like the smile of the Cheshire cat. The metaphoric "sickness" of the mind, under hundreds of names, becomes a hypostatized concept, an "it," which has as much real existence as "god" in heaven, or "love" in the human heart. Three hundred years ago, love was still considered an "illness" (*morbus amoris*), and, provided one keeps to its metaphorical sense, there's a grain of truth in it. It would not even be surprising if some biochemists discovered that people experiencing *amour fou* have a "pink spot" in their urine or any other of the "abnormalities" discovered during the past forty years in "mental" patients (Skrabanek, 1984; 1990).

The purpose of studying human behaviour, whether normal or abnormal, is not to find its correlates in the brain or its "cause" in the genes, but to interpret the *meaning* within the ambit of human relationships. The required discourse is that of the social sciences (which includes psychology) and not that of the biological sciences. It is absurd to study "mental" diseases in animal models, since human behaviour is inseparable from language and symbolic representations. The "winks" of humans cannot be elucidated by pharmacologically induced "blinks" in animals. Nothing can be learned about human behaviour from behaviourist studies in pigeons, except that, in certain circumstances, man can be forced to respond to stimuli as pigeons do. As W. H. Auden observed, "of course, behaviourism works. So does torture."

The first "psychiatric" disease alleged to demonstrate conclusively that human behaviour is "caused" by a specific genetic and biochemical abnormality was the Lesch-Nyhan syndrome, described in 1964. Yet this disease is not a "mental" disease. The patients present with microcephaly, spasticity, mental retardation, choreoathetosis, torsion dystonia, dysarthria, and other neurological symptoms. In addition, they may be "aggressive" and exhibit the characteristic symptoms of compulsive biting of their lips and fingers. Rats injected with various chemicals into the nigrostriatal area may be induced to bite their own limbs and tails. This mutilatory behaviour is worsened by food deprivation or by concomitant "treatment" with scopolamine. In other words, this kind of "behaviour" is similar to other observed behaviours in animals, such as rotatory movement , or "wet-long shakes," which can be induced chemically. It is unlikely that the "self-mutilatory" behaviour of patients with Lesch-Nyhan syndrome is a wilful act, with a symbolic meaning; in other words, it is not an example of *human* behaviour, but rather a primitive reaction, akin to the head-banging of brain-damaged children, tardive diskinesia induced by neuroleptics in psychiatric patients, or floccillation (fitful plucking at bed-clothes) in delirious patients. These are not "behaviours" which can throw light on the mechanism and meaning of "mental" disease or justify inferences that mental disease is "caused" by genes.

Even Roth admits that, "of course, if illness is a matter of lumps, lesions and genes, most schizophrenics are perfectly healthy" (Roth, 1976). So do they, or do they not, have a yet undiscovered brain disease?

What is schizophrenia?

If you talk to God, you are praying; if God talks to you, you have schizophrenia. (Szasz)

Eugen Bleuler, who coined the term "schizophrenia" in 1911, used it as shorthand for "the group of schizophrenias." His son, Manfred, stated that "we are forced to conclude that no single specific cause for all schizophrenic psychoses has been found. I think it does not exist." (Bleuler, 1963). He insisted on treating schizophrenics as moral agents: since there is no specific treatment, the management should "utilise just the same influences [used] in developing and strengthening the healthy: steady human relationship and confrontation with responsibility and danger" (Bleuler, 1968). The Ninth International Classification of Diseases of the W.H.O. (1977) has no entry for "schizophrenia" but rather for a " group of psychoses," known as "schizophrenic psychoses."

Despite enormous efforts and expense (about $100 million a year are spent on schizophrenia research in the United States annually), no specific, objective test for schizophrenia has been discovered. Sarbin (1990) reported that thirty years of psychological research has failed to identify a reliable diagnostic marker which would separate the "schizophrenic" from the non-schizophrenic or the normal. Many psychiatrists are aware of the fact that "there is no clearly delimitable disease entity of schizophrenia with constant causes, psychological picture, or course" (Ciompi, 1984). Among the numerous definitions of "schizophrenia," "there is little evidence that any definition is more valid than another, if indeed any one is valid" (Murray et al., 1985). One set of characteristic features of "schizophrenia" (hallucinations, delusions, etc.), known as Schneider's first-rank symptoms, and thought particularly valuable in distinguishing between schizophrenia and manic-depressive illness or normality, is seen by other respectable researchers as "not schizophrenia" (Kety, 1980). There is no doubt that the concept of schizophrenia has no scientific validity (Boyle, 1990; Sarbin, 1990), yet the term continues to be used in the psychiatric literature as if describing a "disease," rather than serving as an umbrella for a most varied range of behaviours. The diagnosis of schizophrenia becomes a certificate of its existence; it not only explains but it also justifies it.

An English "schizophrenic" is not necessarily labelled as such in France, and vice versa. A questionnaire survey carried out among French and British psychiatrists, consisting of 38 statements about schizophrenia (causation, diagnosis, treatment, prognosis), elicited significant disagreement on 31 statements (van Os et al., 1993). Depending on who is holding the nosological kaleidoscope, different schizophrenic patterns appear. Without being able to maintain schizophrenia as a defined variable, no research on its "causes" is possible. What is the purpose of the most detailed biochemical analysis of brain tissue when the alleged effect, that is, "mental disease," escapes any objective description?

As schizophrenia, by definition, is a non-organic psychosis, then a typical schizophrenic behaviour encountered in various brain disorders, for example, in Huntington's chorea, is not schizophrenia but a schizophreniform symptom of an underlying disease. However, it does not follow that because the cause of Huntington's chorea is a gene defect on chromosome 4, therefore schizophrenia is "caused" by this genetic defect; since schizophrenia is not a definable phenotype. The fact that Huntington's chorea often presents with abnormal behaviour, classifiable under a variety of psychiatric labels (Caine & Shoulston, 1983), should give pause to anyone who searches for causes of mental disease in single genes.

The other major psychosis, besides schizophrenia, is manic-depressive illness. Yet there are no objective criteria by which it may be distinguished. "Whether specific symptoms reliably demarcate the group of illnesses labelled as schizophrenic from manic-depressive illness, that other major group of functional psychoses, on the one hand, and the organic states on the other, are questions which academic psychiatrists continue to debate" (Crow, 1984). This is reminiscent of the medieval debates about the number of angels that can dance on the head of a pin. In a discipline struggling with the "lack of a clear differentiation between normal and abnormal states" (Michels & Marzuk, 1993), it is premature to make assumptions about biological "causes" of such states.

One of the dubious arguments that schizophrenia must be a disease is epidemiological, as schizophrenia is said to occur "at approximately the same incidence in India, Africa, Asia, Europe, and the Americas" (Roth, 1976). How does one diagnose schizophrenia in a !Kung bushman? Through what interpreter? Is the disease occurring with the same incidence among psychiatrists? Aren't genetic diseases characterized by unequal distribution?

If "manic-depressive illness" is a "disease," what is one to make of the statement that "manic-depressive illness often occurs in conjunction with extraordinary talent, even genius, in politics and military leadership, as well as in literature and music and other performing arts" (Gershon & Rieder, 1992)? Should it be "treated" only in those who do not rise through the ranks to become generals? How could the same biochemical (or neuropathological or genetic) abnormality cause insanity in one person and in another, genius?

Psychiatric epidemiologists claim that the life-time prevalence of any mental disorder in the general population of the United States is 33 percent (Michels & Marzuk, 1993). In other words, every family has at least one member who qualifies for psychiatric labelling. *Cui bono?*

Psychopathy - "Sane" insanity?

In 1993, when nurse Beverly Allitt was charged with murdering or attempting to murder 13 children under her care, a forensic psychiatrist diagnosed her as suffering from a "psychopathic disorder," meaning that she had no mental disease, thus allowing the judge to sentence her to 13 life sentences (*Independent*, May 29, 1993). Another expert, Professor Roy Meadow, who was the first to describe "Munchhausen syndrome by proxy," believed that Allitt suffered from this syndrome and that her "condition" could be altered by "therapy." This is the kind of explanation which Peter Medawar called "analgesic," in that it dulls the ache of incomprehension without removing its cause. A general practitioner, together with many ordinary people, thought that Allitt's crimes were so "rare, bizarre and awful as to be almost beyond the imaginings of any sane mind" (*Independent*, May 30, 1993). Yet, according to psychiatrists, she had no mental illness. If "mental illness" has any meaning, then Allitt's mind was as "sick" as it ever can be.

"Psychopathy" is an excellent test case of psychiatric reasoning. The term means literally "sick mind," that is "mental illness," yet its distinctive feature is the absence of mental illness. Psychiatrists are of two minds on this condition. Since psychopathy is not a disease, there is no treatment for it. However, the legal definition of psychopathy requires that it is treatable, so that psychopaths can be involuntarily hospitalized as "criminally insane." According to the 1959 Mental Health Act (England and Wales), psychopathy is a "persistent disorder or disability of mind (whether or not including subnormality of intelligence), which results in abnormally aggressive or seriously irresponsible conduct on the part of the patient and requires, or is susceptible to, medical treatment." Note the terms, "disorder," "disability," "abnormally," "patient," and "treatment." The person labelled as a psychopath is at the same time legally responsible for his "irresponsible conduct" while suffering from a mental "disorder" that can be treated but is not a "disease."

From the point of view of biological psychiatry, "as is the case in the aetiological considerations of most psychiatric conditions, psychopathic personality is in all probability the final common pathway reflecting the interaction of genetic, environmental, biochemical, electrophysiological and endocrine factors" (Rollin, 1975). This seems to cover the whole lot.

As psychopathy is a "disorder of behaviour and socialisation" (Chiswick, 1987) — a description equally fitting any mental disorder — it overlaps, or is synonymous with, "anti-social behaviour," defined as "any deviation from accepted social conventions ... generally in the absence of mental disorder" (Cloninger, 1987). The absence of any brain disease, however, does not stop biological psychiatrists from medicalizing deviant behaviour. Cloninger separates psychopaths (or sociopaths, used synonymously) into seven "syndromes," ranging from a "fretful aggressive" to a "simple extrovert." The latter category includes "successful confidence men." The fretful aggressives are candidates for "treatment" with lithium and neuroleptics; the "hyperkinetic bullies," with pemoline or lithium; and the simple extroverts, with neuroleptics. "Non-aggressive antisocials ... may be treated with the same drugs." In other words, people who do not have a bona fide mental disease are treated with drugs believed to be "specific" for mental diseases.

"The psychopath makes nonsense of every attempt to distinguish the sick from the healthy delinquent by the presence or absence of a psychiatric syndrome, or by syndromes of mental disorder which are independent of his objectionable behaviour. In his case, no such symptoms can be diagnosed because it is just the absence of them which causes him to be classed as psychopathic. He is, in fact, *par excellence*, and without shame or qualification, the model of the circular process by which anti-social behaviour is explained by mental abnormality" (Wooton, 1967). This tautological quandary finds its pseudo-solution in the reductionism of biological psychiatry. All behaviour, in the last analysis, is reducible to brain events, which in turn are generally predetermined. Moral agency is a fiction of moralists.

Meanwhile, psychopaths are "treated" in special hospitals, behind locked doors. Only publicized scandals give the wider public a glimpse of what goes on there. Whistleblowers are rarely psychiatrists themselves, which indicates that gross abuses of power are connived at by the profession. In 1992, for example, Ashworth special hospital (near Liverpool) was described as a "prime candidate to be visited by the European Committee for Prevention of Torture and Inhuman or Degrading Treatment or Punishment" (*Times*, Aug. 6, 1992). Only one among 26 medical staff showed courage to join another 4 complainers (3 psychologists, 1 social worker) who exposed the scandalous treatment of the inmates. Despite a public inquiry and a 400-page report damning the hospital, one year later yet another scandal erupted in the same hospital, this time in the female wing, where anti-psychotic drugs were used as chemical straitjackets, in doses far exceeding the recommended dosage and without psychiatric indication. A professor of clinical pharmacology, Malcolm Lader, testified that in Britain "these drugs probably kill one patient every two weeks" (Dillner, 1993).

The "treatment" may include electroconvulsive therapy (ECT) without anaesthesia. In 1980, when it was discovered that unmodified ECT was used in Broadmoor special hospital to "control" behaviour, it was defended by the President of the Royal College of Psychiatrists and others (*Lancet*, 1980; Crammer, 1980). Perhaps because of inhibitions against soiling one's nest, psychiatrists themselves remain silent, and protest against films such as *One Flew over the Cuckoo's Nest*.

Follies of biological psychiatry

It is not advances in neurophysiology or neurochemistry that shape fashions in psychiatric ontology and epistemology, but the lack of a solid foundation of the discipline. On the one hand, psychiatry wishes to emulate science and escape its metaphysical predicament, while, on the other hand, it also maintains its prerogative to act as a controller of social deviance. Whether psychotherapy (known as "moral treatment" in the past) or somatic treatment predominates as the ruling paradigm depends less on therapeutic results than on the dominant ideology of the profession.

Moral treatment in the York retreat, in the first half of the nineteenth century, was probably as effective as modem biological approaches: about 70 percent of the retreat's patients became well enough to be discharged (Sterling, 1978). This was true when places for the treatment of mental patients were small and staff-patient ratios were high. The success of the Gheel colony, over centuries, can be attributed to this emphasis on a close relationship between the patient and the therapist. With the rise of mammoth asylums, housing up to 10,000 inmates, in appalling conditions, the cure rate plummeted. In the

1930s, with the rise of totalitarianism in Europe and elsewhere, inhuman experimentation with electric shock and psychosurgery on involuntary, captive patients in public asylums became politically and morally acceptable, and the pseudoscience of the leaders of the assault on the brain (Sakel, Meduna, Cerletti, Moniz, Freedman) poisoned the minds of a whole generation of psychiatrists (Skrabanek, 1986; Valenstein, 1986).

The introduction of new psychotropic drugs in the 1950s has been credited with making "deinstitutionalization" possible for the first time. Yet, as Shepherd (1993) pointed out, in hospitals with favorable milieu, psychotropic drugs, despite claims to their "specificity," had little or no effect on discharge rates.

A renewed interest in psychosurgery in the late 1960s was the result of a shifting emphasis from individualized psychiatric care to the control of social deviance, political dissent, urban violence, and drug use (Sterling, 1978; Breggin, 1975; 1983). Evidence for the role of psychosurgery in controlling antisocial behaviour is scientifically worthless (O'Callaghan & Carroll, 1987), but that has been an insufficient reason for not using it. Rather surprisingly, the world leader in psychosurgery is Britain, where it is used especially in "neurosis." Since "there is no objective test for any form of psychiatric illness, the selection for psychosurgery remains a clinical process," Paul Bridges, the chief psychiatrist in the psychosurgical unit at Brook Hospital in London disarmingly admits (Bridges, 1984). The operation consists of destroying normal brain tissue, and the rationale behind this procedure is similar to that of cutting off thieves' hands.

To assault a normal brain with electric current, icepicks (Fredman's method), cryosurgery, cautery, radioactive implants, or a battery of chemicals, because of an *idée fixe* that it is not normal, is more than question-begging — it is more like a symptom of obsessive and delusional thoughts.

The faulty logic of biological psychiatrists can be illustrated by arguments justifying the biological approach, provided by S. Barondes, chairman of psychiatry at the University of California, San Francisco:

since dementia in tertiary syphilis is caused by *Treponema palladium*; depression in myxedema by the lack of thyroxine; impaired intellect in phenylketonuria by a genetic defect; and dementia and expression in pellagra by the lack of niacin, *ergo*, mental diseases have as yet undiscovered structural, chemical, physical, or genetic "causes" (Barondes, 1990). This is a *non-sequitur* on a par with saying that because cats have four legs and dogs have four legs, therefore, cats are dogs. Samuel B. Guze, similarly, believes, that "the best way of conceptualizing psychiatric disorders is to pattern our approach after that used in general medicine," since it is "so successful in the rest of medicine" (Guze, 1991). This reasoning is as sound as that of a man who lost a wallet and was looking for it under a street lamp, not because he lost it there but because that was where the light was.

The 1990s were declared by the U.S. Congress and President Bush as the "Decade of the Brain." In imitation of the search for the Holy Grail of geneticists — mapping of the human genome — the Human Brain Project will "seek to define the structure and function of the last major biological frontier—how we think, create, improvise, learn, how do diseases cause dementia, mania, memory loss, hallucination and delusions" (Cotton, 1993b). Psychiatrists are promised that soon they will be able to say which behaviour is "embedded" in what part of the brain, as if that "enchanted loom where millions of flashing shuttles weave a dissolving pattern" (as C. S. Sherrington described the brain's neuronal net) was some kind of clockwork. We are back to phrenology and locationism. Since the technical language of neurosciences used by biological psychiatrists may dazzle the unwary, it may be salutary to remember that phrenology was accepted as a science by such eminent minds as Augustine Comte, Karl Marx, Goethe, and the editor of the *Lancet*, Thomas Wakely.

The drawing of the brain map is estimated to cost $3 billion. The utopianism of the brain cartographers surpasses even the view of the Council on Long Range Planning and Development of the American Medical Association (1990), who are confident that "studies of positron emission tomography and single-photon emission computed tomographic scans will aid future understanding of schizophrenia, affective disorders, obsessive-compulsive disorder and panic disorder." The Chairman of Psychiatry at Cornell University, Robert Michels, envisages how the psychiatrist of the future will send the patient to have his brain examined by computerized axial tomography, positron emission tomography, and magnetic resonance imaging, for "three-dimensional images of brain structure, density, metabolic activity and chemical composition" (Michels & Markowitz, 1990). There would not be much point in asking the patient any questions, as his thoughts could be directly observed and their density and chemical composition assayed. As Barondes announced, "the psychiatrists and biologists who are committed to a molecular approach to mental illness can confidently look forward to some very productive years" (Barondes, 1990).

The dopamine hypothesis — the mainstay of the biochemical "understanding" of schizophrenia and of its chemical "treatment" — is now in ruins (Waddington, 1993). The effect of neuroleptics upon the "negative" or "defect" symptoms of schizophrenia, which many see as the greatest handicap of such patients, is unclear, as neuroleptics may either improve or exacerbate them (Johnstone, 1993). Biochemical theories, based on the response to chemical manipulation, put the cart before the horse. Because the use of neurochemical agents has been "effective" in psychopaths or political dissidents (one of the reasons for their use), it does not follow that political dissent or psychopathy has a biochemical cause. If the resistance of a Jehovah's Witness to a transfusion can be overcome with a high dose of phenothiazine, it does not follow that an irrational belief about God's prohibition of blood products is due to dopamine hyperactivity.

Psychiatry and genetics

> When little is known in medicine, heredity is invoked as a cause. (J. Jastrow, 1936)

The lure of a genetic "explanation" for crime, alcoholism, homosexuality, drug use, violence, or mental illness is two-fold. For controllers of social deviance it provides a justification for behavioural control with chemicals, brain surgery, or eugenic programs, and for victims it offers exculpation for their transgressions. Moreover, simple explanations for complex problems have an irresistible appeal. A sin and its absolution are entwined in DNA's double helix.

That temperaments, aptitudes, or talents are determined in part by one's genetic endowment has been known for centuries. That certain traits can be enhanced by selective mating has been known by animal breeders also for centuries. However, even simple behavioural patterns in laboratory animals are not dependent on single genes, and most behavioural variability is not genetic in origin (Plomin, 1990). Since genes code for proteins or enzymes and not for psychiatric labels, the matter of psychiatric genetics could be laid to rest here. The recent upsurge in studies purporting to locate a gene for schizophrenia and other mental diseases is more ideologically motivated than the researchers themselves may realize.

Genetic predisposition, or "susceptibility," can always be invoked, even in conditions whose cause is well understood. Not every person exposed to *Mycobacterium tuberculosis* contracts the disease, but in clinical medicine, speculations about the susceptibility to tuberculosis have no practical value since clinical management does not depend on it.

Statements that schizophrenia has a multifactorial and polygenetic aetiology, in which unknown environmental and unknown genetic factors give rise to the clinical manifestation of the disease, have no informational content. The belief that schizophrenia is a genetic disorder is a neo-Lombrosian notion. Sterilization of the "insane" was openly advocated by American psychiatrists from the beginning of the century and as late as 1951 (Gamble, 1951). The involvement of Nazi psychiatrists in the sterilization and "euthanasia" of mental patients is well known. One of the main proponents of the idea that schizophrenia is a genetic disorder was Franz Kallman, who, ironically, as a Jew had to leave Germany in 1936. On his arrival in the United States, he was soon elevated to the position of President of the American Society of

Human Genetics. Kallmann's claims that the concordance rate for schizophrenia between monozygotic twins was 86.2 percent (and 100 percent when "schizoid personality" was included!) (Kallmann, 1953) were eagerly accepted and widely quoted in the psychiatric literature. It is embarrassing to read reviews in the American and British literature unashamedly citing Nazi pseudoscientific research as evidence for the genetic theory.

The concordance rate for schizophrenia between monozygotic twins has been gradually dwindling, as the quality of such studies has improved (Boyle, 1990). Since, even in the most optimistic studies, the concordance rate is less than 50 percent, it is clear that environmental influences are more important than the alleged genetic predisposition. (The concordance rate for crime in monozygotic twins is claimed to be higher than 50 percent [Mednick et al., 1987], but not many psychiatrists would have the courage of their convictions and state openly that criminality is inherited.) An ingenious ad hoc attempt to explain why the majority of monozygotic twins are discordant for schizophrenia is the claim that the asymptomatic twin has a *forme fruste* of the disease, that is, no disease.

Serious methodological and conceptual problems make the evaluation of family and adoption studies difficult (Rose et al., 1984; Lidz & Blatt, 1983; Boyle, 1990), and even biological psychiatrists admit that such studies may be "misleading" (Gurling, 1990).

Thus, when it was announced in national newspapers in the summer of 1988 that "British scientists believe that they pinpointed the location of the gene which causes schizophrenia" (*Observer*, July 24, 1988), there was great excitement all around. The study was published in *Nature* in November (Sherrington et al., 1988). Despite its claim that this was "the first concrete evidence for a genetic basis to schizophrenia," the editor of *Nature* published the study back-to-back with another, which failed to confirm the finding. (*Nature* did it once before in the case of the preposterous homeopathic claim).

Sherrington's study, far from providing evidence that schizophrenia has a genetic basis, presented a paradoxical finding, that when more unspecific diagnosis in the studied families was included (such as depression, alcoholism, drug abuse, phobias, and "other" psychiatric disorders), the linkage to chromosome 5 became better. Serious methodological problems and textual discrepancies in this study were highlighted by Watt and Edwards (1991). When Sherrington's results were presented at a CIBA symposium by the leader of the group, Hugh Gurling, the geneticists who were present were unimpressed. A. G. Motulsky suggested that the term schizophrenia is as vague as "anaemia." Even if a marker gene existed in one particular family, genes still may be of no relevance for the rest of "schizophrenias." To which Gurling replied, "there are only 100,000 genes in the human genome, and therefore many genetic effects on behaviour may be due to single major loci, if, say, half of these genes are encoding proteins for the brain, which is quite possible. Then there will be many genes that cause many phenotypes, and we are just at the beginning of understanding this" (Gurling, 1990). Whether this is a beginning or the end is a moot point, but the employment of genetic psychiatrists is guaranteed for decades ahead.

While the refutation of the idea that schizophrenia is caused by a gene happened instantaneously, in the same issue of *Nature*, the refutation of the claim that bipolar affective disorder is linked to the X chromosome (Xq28 — the same location as the putative marker for homosexuality!) has taken many years (Pauls, 1993).

While it is possible, or even likely, that genes play some role in behavioural patterns, perhaps hundreds of genes, each with a small effect, in a unique combination for each individual, may contribute to personality traits and cognitive abilities (Plomin, 1990). Since the search for such genes is like trying to find not one, but many, needles in the proverbial haystack, the question remains: What would be the purpose of such research, when the effect of environment is, ultimately, the determining factor? No reliable genetic test for schizophrenia is possible, since the presence of many markers would not allow a prediction of who will develop the clinical disease. Why is genetic research of such vital importance to psychiatrists? Only in Utopia will it be possible to replace the whole genome to create a new man in the psychiatrist's image.

A brave new world

In *King Lear*, Gloucester's son Edmond challenges his father's belief that man's fate is predetermined: "That is the excellent foppery of the world that, when we are sick in fortune — often the surfeit of our own behaviour — we make guilty of our disasters the sun, the moon, and the stars; as if we were villains by necessity, fools by heavenly compulsion." Modern psychiatrists have exchanged astrologers' telescopes for geneticists' microscopes.

"I pray that we shall find a specific genetic cause for schizophrenia, for then we may hope that something elective will be done in its prevention," was one psychiatrist's pious wish (Alanen, 1970), who had forgotten "effective" measures enacted in the United States, Scandinavia, and Nazi Germany. Elliot Gershon, who heads the neurogenetics branch of the National Institute of Mental Health, together with the psychiatrist Ronald Rieder, envisages the development of "precise diagnostic tests for persons at risk for (mental) illness, treatments based on knowledge of molecular alterations that lead to illness ... and eventually, the development of gene therapy" (Gershon and Rieder, 1992). Sherrington et al. (1988) were hopeful that "it may eventually be possible for psychiatrists to consider genetic counselling in families where chromosome 5 linkage can be reliably established." That is, "susceptibility" as opposed to disease would be a sufficient reason for taking "effective" measures. The instant reaction to the news that homosexuality is a genetic disorder (unconfirmed, as all other such claims) by the ex-chief rabbi in Britain, Lord Jacobovits, was as follows: "Homosexuality is a disability [his euphemism for "abomination"] and if people wish to have it eliminated before they have children — because they wish to have grandchildren or for other reasons — I do not see any moral objections for using genetic engineering to limit this particular trend" (*Guardian*, June 27, 1993). With a green light from the moralists, supported by more shoddy research, the road will be clear for "effective measures."

The director of the National Institute of Mental Health, psychiatrist Frederick Goodwin, in 1992 launched a campaign to screen children for genetic and biochemical "predisposition" to violence and crime. In his address to the National Health Advisory Council (quoted by Breggin and Breggin, 1993), Goodwin compared inner-city blacks to hyper-aggressive monkeys: "If you look, for example, at male monkeys, especially in the wild, roughly half of them survive to adulthood. The other half die by violence. That is the natural way of it for males, to knock each other off and, in fact, there are some interesting evolutionary implications of that because the same hyper-aggressive monkeys who kill each other are also hypersexual, so they copulate more and therefore reproduce more to offset the fact that half of them are dying." The use of psychosurgery to control antisocial behaviour has been supported by pseudoscientific research on amygdalectomized monkeys (O'Callaghan & Carroll, 1987).

The Lombrosian school of criminal anthropology believed that criminal "stigmata" were evidence of simian ancestry. Animal research is still used as the source of theories for human behaviour. One of the latest lines of research into human violence is the study of genetically engineered mice who lack the serotonin 1B-receptor. "When male mice missing the gene were subjected to a test in which the mouse is isolated for 4 weeks and then faced with an intruder to its cage, they attack the hapless visitor with twice the vigour of a normal mouse" (Barinaga, 1993). Is this to explain why some involuntary patients attack their jailers?

Lewontin (1993), in his spirited attack on the genetic "wonder-workers" and their disciples, who include the editor of *Science*, ridiculed their "visions of genes for alcoholism, unemployment, domestic and social violence and drug addiction. What we have previously imagined to be messy moral, political, and economic issues turn out, after all, to be simply a matter of an occasional nucleotide substitution."

Free will, according to some of these dreamers "is merely a rationalization, artifact or epiphenomenon of biochemical and genetic predestination" — a view dubbed by Cotton (1993a) as neuro-Calvinism. By studying a person's genome, the psychiatrist will be able to predict what the person will do, unless restrained. The director of the U.S. Office of Disease Prevention and Health Promotion predicted that by the year 2000, most people would have their genetic profile on record (Nelkin & Tancredi, 1989). The geneticist Marjory Shaw (1984) proposed that the power of the state should be used to control the spread of genes causing severe deleterious effects, "just as disabling pathological bacteria or viruses are controlled." Blueprints for health fascism are already drawn: the fact that they are based on pseudoscience makes the threat even more ominous.

Conclusions

Many people harbour irrational, bizarre, or crazy ideas, and act in strange ways. This does not make their minds "diseased" in the sense that their behaviour is a disease as any other. Even if an underlying brain disease were to be discovered as the cause of abnormal behaviour, such behaviour would still not be a "disease" but only a symptom, just as cough or fever are not diseases per se, but symptoms of underlying pathology.

Undeterred by a century of vain efforts to find the "cause" of "mental disease" in the brain, biological psychiatrists continue to assault the brain with physical, surgical, or chemical means — a behaviour that can only be described as obsessive or delusional. Yet, the brain is no more "responsible" for the meaning of one's thoughts or acts than a typewriter is for the variety of texts that issue from it. The belief that the mind is reducible to brain events leads to the ultimate neuro-Calvinist absurdity, that man has no free will. The implicit ideology of biological psychiatry is utopian totalitarianism: show me a man's genome and I shall tell you what his mind is; let me manipulate his genes and I shall create a "normal" man-automaton. The door to psycho-eugenics is wide open.

It is essential to keep "what is" separate from "what ought to be." Why people behave in unusual ways, in the absence of a brain disease, is a legitimate subject for psychological inquiry, which cannot be reduced to molecular biology. How society should protect itself against individuals who are dangerous is not a scientific issue, but a political, legal, and ethical problem.

While mental suffering may be harder to bear than somatic complaints, it does not follow that caring for mentally disturbed people, however praise-worthy in its empathy toward others, can be meaningfully described as "treatment" of a disease. When such treatment is administered against the will of the person, who has not sought help, it can only be described as assault and battery. The dual role of psychiatrists, willingly accepted and cherished, as carers and jailers, as counsellors and soul-destroyers, accounts for the chronically sick state of the discipline.

References

Alanen YO. The families of schizophrenic patients. *Proceedings of the Royal Society of Medicine* 1970; 63: 22-231.

Anon. ECT in Broadmoor. *Lancet* 1980; i: 348-349.

Baringa M. The mice that roared. *Science* 1993; 262: 1211.

Barondes SH. The biological approach to psychiatry: history and prospects. *Journal of Neuroscience* 1990; 10: 1707-1710.

Bleuler M. Conception of schizophrenia within the last fifty years and today. *Proceedings of the Royal Society of Medicine* 1963; 56: 945-952.

Bleuler M. A 23-year longitudinal study of 208 schizophrenics and impressions in regards to the nature of schizophrenia. In: Rosenthal D and Kety SS. eds.The Transmission of Schizophrenia. Pergamon Press, New York, 1968

Boyle M. Schizophrenia: A Scientific Delusion? Routledge, London, 1990

Breggin PR. Psychosurgery for political purposes.
Duquesne Law Review 1975; 13: 841-862.

Breggin PR. The return of lobotomy and psychosurgery. In: Edwards RB ed.

Psychiatry and Ethics. Prometheus Books, New York, 1983:350-388.

Breggin PR and Breggin GR. A biomedical programme for urban violence control in the US: the dangers of psychiatric social control. *Changes* 1993; 11: 59-71.

Bridges PK. Psychosurgery and the Mental Health Commission. *Bulletin of the Royal College of Psychiatry* 1984; 8: 146-148.

Caine ED and Shoulston I. Psychiatric syndromes in Huntington's disease. *American Journal of Psychiatry* 1983; 140: 728-733.

Chiswick D. Managing psychopathic offenders: a problem that will not go away. *British Medical Journal* 1987; 295: 159-190.

Ciompi L. Is there really a schizophrenia? The long-term course of psychotic phenomena. *British Journal of Psychiatry* 1984; 145: 636-640.

Cloninger C R . Pharmacological approaches to the treatment of anti-social behavior. In: Mednik SA, Moffit TE, Stack SA eds. The Causes of Crime — New Biological Approaches. Cambridge University Press, Cambridge, 1987: 329-349.

Cotton P. Neurophysiology, philosophy on collision course? *Journal of the American Medical Association* 1993; 269: 1485-1486.(a)

Cotton P. Scientists chart course for brain map. *Journal of the American Medical Association* 1993; 269: 1357(b)

Council on Long Range Planning and Development. The future of psychiatry. *Journal of the American Medical Association* 1990; 264: 2542-2548.

Crammer J. Unmodified ECT. *Lancet* 1980; i: 486.

Crow T J. Schizophrenia — the problem of the mechanism of the disturbance and its causation. In: Duncan R and Weston-Smith M eds.The Encyclopædia of Medical Ignorance. London: Pergamon Press, London, 1984.

Dillner L. Inquiry says depot injections can kill. *British Medical Journal* 1993; 307: 641.

Gamble CJ. Sterilization in preventive psychiatry. *American Journal of Psychiatry* 1951; 107: 932-934.

Gershon ES and Rieder RO. Major disorders of mind and brain.

Scientific American 1992; 266: 127-133.

Gurling HMD. (1990). Recent advances in genetics of psychiatric disorders. In: Human Genetic Information: Science, Law and Ethic (CIBA Foundations Symposium 149). Wiley, Chichester, 1990: 48-62.

Guze SB. What is psychiatry? *Biological Psychiatry* 1991; 29: 1156-1160.

Johnstone EC. Schizophrenia: problems in clinical practice. *Lancet* 1993; 341: 536-538.

Kallmann FJ. Heredity in Health and Mental Disorder. Principles of Psychiatric Genetics in the Light of Comparative Twin Studies. Norton & Co, New York, 1953.

Kety SS. The syndrome of schizophrenia: unresolved questions and opportunities for research. *British Journal of Psychiatry* 1990; 136: 421-436.

Leifer R. Psychiatry, language and freedom. *Metamedicine* 1982; 3: 397-416.

Lewontin R. The Doctrine of DNA. Biology as Ideology. Penguin Books, Harmondsworth, 1993.

Lidz T and Blatt S. Critique of the Danish-American studies of the biological and adaptive relatives of adoptees who become schizophrenic. *American Journal of Psychiatry* 1983; 140: 426-434.

Mednick SA, Moffitt TE and Stack SA eds. The Causes of Crime. New Biological Approaches. Cambridge University Press, Cambridge, 1987.

Michels R and Markowitz JC. The future of psychiatry. *Journal of Medical Philosophy* 1990; 15: 5-9.

Michels R and Marzuk PM. Progress in psychiatry. *New England Journal of Medicine* 1993; 329: 552-560.

Murray RM, Lewis SW and Reveley AM. Towards an aetiological classification of schizophrenia. *Lancet* 1985; i: 1023-1026.

Nelkin D.and Tancredi L. Dangerous Diagnostics. The Social Power of Biological Information. Basic Books, New York, 1989.

O'Callaghan MAJ and Carroll D. The role of psychosurgical studies in the control of anti-social behavior. In: Mednick SA, Moffitt TE, Stack SA.eds.The Causes of Crime. New Biological Approaches. Cambridge University Press,

Cambridge, 1987: 312-328.

Pauls DL. Behavioural disorders: lessons in linkage.
Nature Genetics 1993; 3: 4-5.

Plomin R. The role of inheritance in behaviour. *Science* 1990; 248: 183-188.

Popper KR. Objective Knowledge. An Evolutionary Approach. Clarendon Press, Oxford, 1972: 206-265.

Popper KR and Eccles JC. The Self and Its Brain. Springer International, New York, 1978.

Rollin HR. Psychological medicine: personality disorders.
British Journal of Medicine 1975; 1: 665-667.

Rose S. Molecules and Minds: Essays on Biology and Social Order. Open University Press, Milton Keynes, 1987.

Roth M. Schizophrenia and the theories of Thomas Szasz.
British Journal of Psychiatry 1976; 129: 317-326.

Sarbin TR. Towards the obsolescence of the schizophrenia hypothesis. *Journal of Mind and Behavior* 1990; 11: 259-283.

Searle J. The Rediscovery of the Mind. Journal of Legal Medicine. MIT Press, Cambridge, 1992.

Shaw MW. Conditional prospective rights of the fetus.
Journal of Legal Medicine 1984; 63: 63-116.

Shepherd M. The placebo: from specificity to the non-specific and back.
Psychological Medicine 1993; 23: 569-578.

Sherrington R, Brynjolfsson J, Petursson H, Potter M, Dudleston K, Barraclough B, Wasmuth J, Dobbs M and Gurling H. Localization of a susceptibility locus for schizophrenia on chromosome 5. *Nature* 1988; 336: 164-167.

Skrabanek P. Biochemistry of schizophrenia: a pseudoscientfic model.
Integrative Psychiatry 1984; 2: 224-236.

Skrabanek P. Convulsive therapy — a critical appraisal of its origins and value. *Irish Medical Journal* 1986; 79: 157-165.

Skrabanek P. Reductionist fallacies in the theory and treatment of mental disorders. *International Journal of Mental Health* 1988; 19(3): 6-18.

Sperry R. Psychologist's mentalist paradigm and the religion/science tension. *American Psychologist* 1988; 43: 607-613.

Sterling P. Ethics and effectiveness of psychosurgery. In: Brady JP and Brodie HKH. Controversy in Psychiatry.
W.B. Saunders Co, Philadelphia, 1978: 126-160.

Valenstein ES. Great and Desperate Cures. The Rise and Decline of Psychosurgery and Other Radical Treatments for Mental Illness. Basic Books, New York, 1986.

Van Os J, Galdos P, Lewis G, Bourgeois M and Mann A. Schizophrenia sans frontiers: concept of schizophrenia among French and British psychiatrists. *British Medical Journal* 1993; 307: 489-492.

Waddington JL. Schizophrenia: developmental neuroscience and pathobiology. *Lancet* 1993; 341: 531-536.

Watt DC and Edwards JH. Doubts about evidence for a schizophrenia gene on chromosome 5. *Psychological Medicine* 1991; 21: 279-285.

Wooton B. Social Science and Social Pathology. Allen & Unwin, 1967.

6

SCEPTICISM, IRRATIONALISM AND PSEUDOSCIENCE

Abstract My course on the critical appraisal of evidence, for medical students, can be compared to a course on miracles by a Humean sceptic for prospective priests in a theological seminary.

Medicine is an authoritarian institution which feels threatened when its dogmas are exposed as a refuge for ignorance. In his Harveian Oration, Sir George Pickering pointed out that "from the time of Galen to our own, medicine has always presented a façade of systematic knowledge, or alleged knowledge, for, like religion, medicine could not tolerate ignorance".[1] Since medicine, unlike religion, aspires to be a science, it is torn by the irreconcilable conflict between the need for criticism and the fear of it. For many medical students the first exposure to this conflict is a disturbing experience.

While the threat of criticism to medicine is largely imaginary, the real threat is posed by uncritical acceptance of principles of 'alternative' medicine. The exploitation of irrational healing methods by the medical profession is on the increase.[2,3] Recently, *The Lancet* announced that three trials of faith healing are underway in British academic institutions, testing the benefits of faith healing in patients with cataract, patients with rheumatoid arthritis, and horses with intestinal parasites.[4] The announcement did not make it clear whether in the last trial it is the worms, the horse, or the investigator whose faith is required.

Today's medicine is defenceless against such travesty of reason, because it lacks criteria for the demarcation of the absurd. It would be

---

This paper was read at the Philosophy Seminar of the Department of Philosophy, Trinity College, on 17 January 1986. A shortened version was published under the title "Demarcation of the absurd" in *The Lancet*, 960-961, 26 April 1986.

naive to presume that 'alternative medicine' is a transient fad which will quickly pass away because it only appeals to fools. In his undeservedly little known *Christian Science*, Mark Twain argued that this is the very reason why it would continue to flourish: "Christian Science is 'restricted' to the unintelligent, the people who do not think. Therein lies the danger. It makes it formidable."[5]

The medical school should teach the student how to winnow the chaff of charlatanism from the wheat of science. This will not be possible before the roots of gullibility have been exposed and cut. At present, the difference between a doctor and a quack is determined not by the nature of their practice but by the possession of a medical diploma.

Karl Popper expressed a similar concern when he wrote about the failure of arts faculties to produce graduates who could distinguish between a charlatan and a scholar.[6] However, he backtracked before the charge of elitism and admitted later that there was a place in science even for the charlatan.[7] The reason for this vacillation is Popper's lack of criteria for demarcating the absurd. However, Popper's admonition to teachers of arts subjects is equally applicable to medical education and science education: "Not only does it fail to educate the student, who is often to become a teacher, to an understanding of the greatest spiritual movement of his day, but it also often fails to educate him to intellectual honesty".[6]

Scepticism and demarcation of the absurd

"The aim of science is not to open a door to infinite wisdom but to set a limit to infinite error", in words of Brecht's Galileo.[8] It is a paradox that scepticism both helps and hinders critical inquiry. As Bevan wrote many years ago, a consistent sceptic is driven to a position in which every dogma might be false and every superstition might be true.[9] This sceptical straw-man would refuse to incant the *Credo quia impossibile* (I believe it because it is impossible), while conceding the *Non nego quia ineptum* (I cannot deny it because it is absurd). The rational sceptic does not fall into this trap. He distinguishes between rational and irrational belief. A 'belief' in the value of rational argument is quite different from a 'belief' in angels. Even the believer in angels believes in the value of rational criticism when it can serve as a defence against nonbelievers or provide new converts. Those who believe in reason are often accused of having a belief that is no better than an irrational belief. This charge is usually brought in when the irrationalist has run out of defensive arguments. It is not 'belief' versus 'scepticism' which distinguishes the rationalist from the irrationalist, but the nature of their beliefs and scepticism. Irrational scepticism is characterized by an inability to accept the existence of the absurd: one's mind stays so open that the brains fall out. Anything is possible. In this way, irrational scepticism is used as a defence mechanism for sanctioning absurd beliefs. It is a protracted suicide of reason. On the other hand, scepticism may stir us from dogmatic slumbers. A rational sceptic shuts his mind in the face of absurdity. He uses a sceptical mode to justify his unbelief. Schematically the dual role of scepticism can be shown as follows:

Scepticism about rationality ⟨ Dogmatic belief (in the absurd)
(irrational scepticism)   Tentative unbelief (in reason)

Scepticism about knowledge, facts ⟨ Dogmatic unbelief (in the absurd)
(rational scepticism)   Tentative belief (in facts)

Irrational scepticism is represented by Descartes, who doubted the obvious and believed the incredible.

Rational scepticism is more an attitude of mind than a philosophy; it is the basis of scientific thinking. Rational sceptics are often labelled as agnostics or atheists—a meaningless distinction, the subtlety of which tickles the fancy of the irrationalists. Rational scepticism is often declared 'dangerous' by religious authorities, because it undermines belief, leaving knowledge uncertain. On the other hand, irrational scepticism is welcomed by authorities as it only undermines rational knowledge but leaves beliefs intact.

Both rational and irrational scepticism should not be confused with philosophical scepticism originating in the teaching of Pyrrho of Elis (360-275 BC). Pyrrho reached his sceptical position not as a result of wishing to know or to believe, but because he thought that the desire to know is futile and leads to unhappiness.[10] He was probably a disillusioned moralist who yearned for a utopia in which reason does not exist, the state of *ataraxia* (i.e. imperturbability) and of *apathia* which filled the mental horizon of Adam and Eve before their first human act—a rational inquiry, an experimental tasting of the fruit from the tree of knowledge.

Of the ancient sceptics perhaps the closest to the position of the modern rational sceptics was Carneades of Cyrene (213-129 BC) and his pupil, Cleitomachus, a Jew from Carthage. Carneades believes that while neither reason nor the senses are infallible, some sense data and some opinions are more likely to be true than others. If data were not contradicted by experience and if they survived critical tests, they became more probable. This sounds surprisingly modern. As could be expected, Carneades' school was attacked by the Neo-Pyrrhonians as 'dogmatic' because they rescinded the Pyrrhonian *isosthenia*, i.e. allowing equal strength to both sides of any argument.[10]

The modern scepticism is usually dated from Descartes. Descartes missed the whole point of rational scepticism by postulating that "in order to investigate the truth of things it is necessary *once in one's life* [my emphasis] to put all things in doubt". After this doubting once he plunged into his new dogmatism, conjuring up a Perfect Being out of thin air. Descartes' *cogito ergo sum* became quickly a target of ridicule from Gassendi to Bayle, as discussed in Popkin's classic.[11] Gassendi (1592-1655) thought that the *cogito* proved nothing and nothing could follow from it. His pupil, Samuel Sorbière, saw it as useless doubting, which led to preposterous affirming. Three hundred years later, Ambrose Bierce summarized the Cartesian starting point as follows: "The *cogito ergo sum*—whereby Descartes was pleased to suppose that he demonstrated the reality of human existence—might be improved as *cogito cogito ergo cogito sum*, i.e. I think that I think, therefore I think that I am—as close an approach to certainty as any philosopher has yet made". [12]

Note that Descartes was attacked by Jesuit sceptical philosophers who accused him of trying to rationalize, and thus subvert, Christianity. The point has a permanent validity. According to Bishop Pierre-Daniel Huet (1630-1721), Christianity was based on faith alone and there should be no rational evidence of God and no rational justification of the truth of Christianity. Paradoxically, this ultrasceptical defence of Christianity by irrational sceptics (in my terminology) was turned upside down in the next century by the French Enlightenment thinkers, who, using the same argument, mounted the sceptical attack on Christianity. David Hume was also aware of the double-edge of the sceptical scalpel. In his essay on miracles, Hume hoped that he had succeeded in confounding "those *dangerous friends* and *disguised enemies* [my emphasis] of the Christian religion who have undertaken to defend it by the principles of human reason".[13]

Whether Pierre Bayle (1647-1706) was a dangerous friend or a disguised enemy is a moot point. Popkin is undecided as to whether Bayle in his massive *Dictionnaire historique et critique* was trying to destroy reason for the sake of religion, or, rather, to destroy religion for the sake of reason.[11] This uncertainty is partially due to the fact, alluded to earlier, that both rationalists and irrationalists have to use rational arguments. As Hume noticed in the Treatise, the enemy of reason is obliged to use rational arguments to prove the fallaciousness and imbecility of reason.[14] However, the rationalist may not use irrational arguments to defeat irrationalism.

Bayle in his eight-million-word dictionary reduced all intellectual pretensions in theology, philosophy and science *ad absurdum*. He advocated, at least on the face of it, the acceptance of faith without reason. Whether with tongue in cheek or not, in note B to *Pyrrho*, Bayle wrote that "the grace of God in the faithful, the force of education in other men, and even, if you wish, ignorance, and the natural inclination to reach decisions, all these constitute an impenetrable shield against the arrows of the Pyrrhonians".[11] This could be rephrased as follows: religion, dogmatic education, ignorance and wishful thinking prevent people from using their reason critically.

Wishful thinking

"Just as we swallow food because we like it and not because of its nutritional content, so do we swallow ideas because we like them and not because of their rational content". [15]

Even great thinkers, such as Descartes, Berkeley, or Newton, could not resist the overpowering pull of their own wishful thinking towards the abyss of the absurd. What made the cool, analytical mind of the creator of Sherlock Holmes believe in fairies and write a book about it?[16] Bishop Berkeley believed that tar water was the closest natural thing to drinkable God and a universal panacea.[17] Lord Bacon confessed that he did not entirely discredit the "weapon-salve" (i.e. an ointment applied not to the wound but to the weapon) for curing wounds. Van Helmont and William Harvey were among those who believed in the curative properties of being touched by the hand of one who died a slow death. Robert Boyle, the President of the Royal Society, believed that he was cured of the ague by wearing a brass bracelet. The first Astronomer Royal, Reverend John Flamsteed, came to Ireland to be touched by the quack Greatrakes. The philosopher Dr David Hartley, who was also a medical doctor, believed that he was cured of stone by a patent remedy: he wrote an adulatory book about the infallible cure with Mrs Stephens's powder, but he died of the disease.[18] Margaret Mead was a fervent believer in the occult and found the evidence for the visits by the UFOs (unidentified flying objects) incontestable. The UFO sighting by Jimmy Carter, which he duly reported, was found to be the planet Venus.[19]

How could the incomparable Isaac Newton write a whole book on the fulfilment of the prophecies of Daniel and the Apocalypse of St John? Newton discovered that the Church of Rome was the eleventh horn of the fourth beast of Daniel's vision, and computed that it would be erased from the Earth between the years 2035 and 2054 (being a mathematician he provided a confidence interval).[20] Sir William Whitla, a professor of the medical faculty at Queen's University in Belfast, and president of the British Medical Association, republished Newton's book in 1922. He warned, in his introduction, against scepticism, atheism, pantheism, deism, agnosticism, materialism and rationalism. He noted that among those who dismissed Biblical miracles were those "who deny such modern discoveries of the psychical research as the fact of levitation". He mentioned with approval "the illustrious Lord Kelvin, who was a devout believer and student of the sacred oracles, and anyone who had heard his opening prayers at the commencement of his daily lecture in the University of Glasgow could never doubt his sincerity".

H.L. Mencken, in a review of a book on science and religion by an eminent Baltimore gynaecologist, Howard Kelly, who believed in Jonah and the whale, asked: "How is it possible for a human brain to be divided into two insulated halves, one functioning normally, naturally, and even brilliantly, and the other capable of ghastly balderdash?"[21]

By considering these examples as deterrents, it is easy to construct rules for avoiding the baneful influence of wishful thinking, but it is extremely difficult to apply them. We know that "we must search our mind beforehand to find out what we would like to be true, and having got that clear, constantly discount our natural tendency in that direction".[22] The more strongly we feel about our opinion, the more likely we hold it on irrational grounds. Unfortunately, these warnings fall on deaf ears, particularly the ears of those who might profit from them most. Critical unbelief, i.e. rational scepticism, is possibly an innate property of mind, rather than a result of education. As Hume noted in the Treatise: "belief is some sensation or peculiar manner of conception, which it is impossible for mere ideas and reflections to destroy".[14]

Recently I was talking to two scientists who believed in homoeopathy. It transpired that they knew next to nothing about the principles of this infinitesimal discipline, but that did not stop them defending it: "you have to keep your mind open". The absurdity of homoeopathy becomes obvious when it is realized that the 'infinitesimal' doses commonly used by the homoeopathists exceed in dilution the Avogadro number. This means that the resultant 'remedy' does not contain even a single molecule of the substance of which it pretends to be a dilution. A dilution of '30C', i.e. 30th centesimal dilution, and a medium dilution by homoeopathic standards, corresponds to a grain of a substance dissolved in a volume sufficient to fill 140 billion spheres, each extending from limit to limit of the Neptune orbit. The gullible patient is invited to gulp down a few drops of these dilutions of grandeur each day. Overdose is dangerous, since, according to the homoeopathists, the more dilute the solution is, the more potent it becomes. Unfortunately, it does not apply for alcohol.[23]

Open mind or open sink?

The absurdity of homoeopathy and other 'alternatives' is usually defended by a 'sceptical' argument that we should keep our mind open, while, at the same time, being exhorted that we must be sceptical about orthodox medicine and its tenets. That certain tenets of orthodox medicine are as vulnerable to rational analysis as those of alternative medicine neither justifies the latter nor condemns the valid content of the former.

The 'open mind' is not a prerogative of irrational sceptics. Professor Paul Kurtz, from the State University of New York and chairman of the Committee for the Scientific Investigation of Claims of the Paranormal, stated: "We can ask, Does sleeping under a pyramid increase sexual potency? Do plants have ESP (extra-sensory perception) and will talking to them enhance their growth? Do tape recorders really pick up voices of the dead? All these claims have been made by paranormalists within the past decade. They should not be rejected out of hand".[24]

By refusing to reject absurd claims out of hand, Kurtz betrays that he lacks a demarcation criterion of the absurd, though he is aware of the necessity of such demarcation: "thus we must keep an open mind . .

. but one should make a distinction between the open mind and open sink".[24]

On the other hand, irrational sceptics find scepticism a useful device to protect their dogmas. Christians, whose religion is based on miracles (such as resurrection, transubstantiation, and divine intervention) sometimes employ scepticism either to reject undesirable miraculous phenomena or to doubt scientific theories. While in August 1985, Cardinal O'Fiaich directed prayers throughout the Armagh diocese for good weather (*The Irish Times*, 28 August, 1985), another representative of the Church, Very Reverend Killian Dwyer, two weeks later, expressed doubts about 'moving statues' observed in several Irish localities and said that the attitude of the Catholic Church to this widespread phenomenon "bordered on the sceptical" (*The Irish Times*, 13 September, 1985). This illustrates that irrational sceptics can maintain a sceptical attitude when convenient, while practising magical thinking.

John MacManners, reviewing a book on the Jansenist convulsionists of St Médard in Paris in the eighteenth century (*Times Literary Supplement*, 26 July, 1985) pointed out that despite the fact that the miracles at St Médard's were attested by thousands of documents and testimonies of eyewitnesses, duly certified by notaries, and authenticated to a far greater degree than the gospel stories, they were held by the Church to be fraudulent.

An interesting example of the ultimate scepticism by a Christian dogmatist is found in a speech in Oxford by John Henry Newman. Trying to reconcile the irreconcilable—the conflict between the Bible and Galileo, he spoke as follows: "Scripture says that the Sun moves and the Earth is stationary, and science that the Earth moves and the Sun is comparatively at rest. How can we determine which of these statements is the very truth till we know what motion is? If our idea of motion is but an accidental result of our present senses, neither proposition is true or both are true; neither is true philosophically; both are true for certain practical purposes".[25] This is an amazing piece of rhetoric. Newman had to know, of course, that the Inquisition put it to Galileo that to claim that the Earth is a Sun's planet was "absurd, philosophically false, and formally heretical, because it expressly contradicted the Holy Scriptures". Newman paid lip-service to the Scriptures lest he appeared heretical, and he bowed to science lest he appeared obscurantist in front of Oxford dons and students. The result was a meaningless statement, yet anticipating unwittingly Einstein's relativism.

The early Christians were not ashamed to admit what they believed as absurd. Tertullian, who lived at the time of the sceptic Sextus Empiricus in the second century, expressed the central dogma of Christianity in his famous formulation: *Crucifixus est dei filius; non pudet, quia pudendum est. Et mortuus est dei filius; prorsus credibile est, quia ineptum est. Et sepultus resurrexit, certum est, quia impossibile.* [26] (The Son of God was crucified; that is not shameful, because it is shameful. And the Son of God died; that is credible, because it is absurd. And He rose from the dead; that is quite certain, because it is impossible.) At least this position is unassailable by reason because it stands outside reason.

Demarcation of the absurd

"No testimony is sufficient to establish a miracle unless the testimony be of such a kind that its falsehood would be (even) more miraculous than the fact which it endeavours to establish".[13] This golden rule should bear the name Hume's Razor. In his *History*, Hume wrote that "it is business of history to distinguish between the miraculous and the marvellous; to reject the first . . . and to doubt the second".[27] Here Hume adopts rational scepticism in advocating dogmatic unbelief in the absurd ('miraculous') and tentative unbelief in the unusual ('marvellous'). The *onus probandi* for unusual claims should rest with the claimant. Hume's rational scepticism was considered by the Church so dangerous that all his works were put on her *Index of Prohibited Books* in 1761; the ban was renewed in 1827 and was still in force in the latest edition of 1948.[28]

Wittgenstein thought that philosophy must set limits to what can be thought, and in doing so, to what cannot be thought. His demarcation criterion was strictly limited to logic: "Just as the only necessity that exists is logical necessity, so too the only impossibility that exists is logical impossibility" (*Tractatus* 6.375). This criterion does not help to distinguish between a charlatan and a scholar, or between a crank and a scientist. A physicist will show the door to a would-be inventor of *perpetuum mobile* without bothering to inspect the 'invention', not because it is logically impossible to construct *perpetuum mobile* but because, in the context of thermodynamics, the proposition is absurd.

Popper's criterion of falsifiability (testability) does demarcate between empirical and metaphysical statements, but is so wide that it allows non-metaphysical nonsense to slip in. A statement such as "In Azerbaijan there lives a man who was born in 1500", with his address and photograph supplied, is clearly absurd, although neither illogical nor untestable. The criterion of falsifiability alone is not sufficient to distinguish a crank from a scientist. The statement "The moon is made of blue cheese", made before the space flights were possible, was metaphysical nonsense; the same statement made at present is empirical nonsense.

Fred Gruenberger proposed the following checklist for screening crackpots: public verifiability, predictability, testability, fruitfulness, Occam's razor, authority, humility, open-mindedness, paranoia, and dollar-complex.[29] Bunge added criteria based on attitudes towards ignorance, problem solving, hypothesis testing, search for laws, cherishing unity of science, reliance on logic, search for counter-examples, settling disputes by experimentation, seeking critical comments, and attitude towards unfavourable data.[30]

In trying to demarcate the absurd, it is as important to know who says what and why, as to know what is being said and how. If a monkey types by accident "I am a monkey", the message is meaningless, despite its apparent truthfulness. Absurdity is contextual.

When in 1905 Einstein postulated that Lorentz's transformations were more than a useful mathematical device but had, in fact, a physical meaning, the consequences appeared absurd to laymen: absolute time had no physical reality; times shown on clocks in motions relative to each other were not synchronous. The article, however, was accepted by the editors of *Annalen der Physik*, and by Einstein's peers, as a significant advance in theoretical physics. Einstein later recalled that "the type of critical reasoning which was required for the discovery of this central point (i.e., the arbitrariness of the concept of simultaneity) was decisively furthered, in my case, especially by reading of David Hume's and Ernst Mach's philosophical writings".[31] Einstein praised in particular "the incorruptible scepticism" of Mach, who did not even believe in the existence of atoms; this did not diminish Mach as a physicist, as his disbelief was not irrational, but merely erroneous. If, on the other hand, Mach believed in miracles, his scientific credibility would be at stake.

For a philosophical sceptic there is always a dilemma how to navigate between the Scylla of gullibility and the Charybdis of disbelief, as if the safe path had to lie in between. This ulyssean analogy is lame: it does not follow that, if the two extreme positions are 2+2=6 and 2+2=4, that truth lies in the middle: 2+2=5. By choosing unbelief, we do not rule out a subsequent change of opinion, based on new evidence, and thus nothing is lost; whereas, by being gullible, we lose reason from the very beginning.

The worst that can happen by following this pragmatic strategy of rational scepticism is that the baby of truth will be thrown out with the absurd bathwater. This analogy, however, is grossly misleading. First, the 'bath' is not a bath but a vast sea of nonsense. Second, it is not one imaginary Gargantuan baby we should worry about but rather the fate of thousands upon thousands of our fellow-men, who, swallowing gallons of water and blindly thrashing in this absurd ocean, are near drowning. We must first rescue them from the teeth of the sharks of untruth and from their watery grave by pulling them ashore. Only then, when they are dry and safe, can we sit together, sample the sea, and, peering down our microscopes, marvel at the immortal plankton of truth.

References

1. Pickering G. Physician and scientist. *Br Med J* 1964; ii: 1615-1619.

2. Reilly DT. Young doctors' views on alternative medicine. *Br Med J* 1983; 287: 337-339.

3. Fulder SJ and Munro RE. Complementary medicine in the U.K.: patients, practitioners, and consultations. *Lancet* 1958; ii, 542-545.

4. Exploring the effectiveness of healing. *Lancet* 1985; ii: 1177-1178 ; *Lancet* 1987; i: 343

5. Twain M. Christian Science. In Raender P ed. Works of Mark Twain. Volume 19, University of California Press, Berkeley, 1973: 263

6. Popper KR. The Open Society and its Enemies. Volume 2, 5th edn. Routledge & Kegan Paul, London, 1965: 283

7. Popper KR. Realism and the Aim of Science. Hutchinson, London, 1985: 70.

8. Bevan E. Stoics and Sceptics. Clarendon Press, Oxford, 1913: 148.

9. Brecht B. Leben des Galilei. Suhrkamp, Berlin, 1963: 85.

10. Bury EG ed. Sextus Empiricus. Introduction. Volume 1. Heinemann, London, 1933.

11. Popkin RH. The High Road to Pyrrhonism. Austin Hill Press, San Diego, 1980.

12. Bierce A. The Devil's Dictionary. Dover, New York, 1958.

13. Hume D. An Inquiry Concerning Human Understanding. Edited by Selby-Bigge LA. Oxford University Press, London, 1902: 115

14. Hume D. A Treatise of Human Nature. Edited by Selby-Bigge LA. Oxford University Press, London, 1906.

15. Jones FA ed. Richard Asher Talking Sense. Pitman, London, 1972.

16. Brandon R. The Spiritualists. Wiedenfeld & Nicolson, London. 1983.

17. Berman D. Bishop Berkeley and the fountains of living waters. *Hermathena* 1980; 128: 21-31.

18 Simpson JY. Homoeopathy: its Tenets and Tendencies. Sutherland & Knox, Edinburgh,1853: 36

19 Gardner M. Margaret Mead and the paranormal.
    Skeptical Inquirer 1983; 8: 13-19.

20 Newton I. Observations upon the Prophecies of Daniel and the Apocalypse of St John. J. Darby and T. Browne, London, 1733.

21 Mencken HL. Prejudices. 6th Series, J. Cape, London, 1928: 154.

22 Crawshay-Williams R. The Comforts of Unreason. A Study of the Motives behind Irrational Thought. Kegan Paul, London, 1947: 43.

23 Skrabanek P. Is homoeopathy a placebo response?
    Lancet 1986; ii: 1107.

24 Kurtz P. Debunking, neutrality, and skepticism in science.
    Skeptical Inquirer 1984; 8: 239-246 .

25 Newman JH. Sermons on the theory of religious belief. Quoted by AD White in A History of the warfare of Science with Theology in Christendom, Volume 2. Cornell University Press, Ithaca, 1895: 166.

26 Tertullian. De carne Christi. Evans E ed. SPCK, London,1956.

27 Hume D. The history of Great Britain from the invasion of Julius Caesar to the Revolution in 1688, Volume 2. Quoted by Flew A. Hume's Philosophy of Belief, Routledge & Kegan Paul, London, 1961:194.

28 Index librorum prohibitorum,Typis Polyglottis Vaticanis, Vatican, 1948: 225.

29 Gruenberger F. A measure for crackpots.
    Science 1964; 145: 1413-1415.

30 Bunge M. What is pseudoscience? *Skeptical Inquirer* 1984; 9: 36-46 .

31 Einstein A. Autobiographical Notes. In Schilpp A ed. Albert Einstein-Philosopher-Scientist, Volume 1, 3rd edn.
    Open Court, La Salle, 1969: 53.

7

CERVICAL CANCER IN NUNS AND PROSTITUTES: A PLEA FOR SCIENTIFIC CONTINENCE

Introduction

An expert answering a reader's query in a medical weekly stated about carcinoma of the cervix that "it is now well documented that the disease is rare in nuns and common in prostitutes", adding, somewhat cryptically, that "a connection between intercourse and cervical cancer was apparently first suggested in 1842" [1]. Both statements are false but widely believed to be true, presumably because they support what is believed to be proved.

Rigoni-Stern, 1842

A reference to an obscure Italian communication from 1842 has become *de rigueur* in the opening paragraphs of articles on the aetiology of cervical cancer, but how many authors have read the original? For example, an early culprit wrote: "Speculation on the relation of marriage to onset of cervical cancer goes back to 1842, when Rigoni-Stern proposed the non-married status of Catholic Sisters as a reason for an associated low frequency" [2]. Subsequent authors, copying from each other, gradually embellished the nun's tale, adding various invented details.

Rigoni-Stern was a Veronese surgeon and an amateur epidemiologist [3]. He analysed over 150,000 death certificates from the Veronese district for the years 1760-1839. Of 74,184 women who died, 1288 were nuns. Rigoni-Stern estimated that cancer in nuns was about five times more common than in other women, mainly because of an excess of breast cancer in nuns. He made no comments on "rarity" of cervical cancer in nuns, as cervical cancer was not distinguished from other cancers of the uterus. In fact, he recorded four deaths from uterine

---

This paper first appeared in the *Journal of Clinical Epidemiology*, Volume 41, No 6, pages 577-582 (1988)

cancer in nuns, while the expected number (based on 361 cases in the remaining 72,896 women) was six. The very low numbers for this and other cancers in Rigoni-Stern's data suggest under-diagnosis [4].

Other nun studies

The evidence for the claim that cervical cancer is rare in nuns rests on the work of Gagnon [5]. He searched "medical files of an annual average of 13,000 women, covering a twenty-year period, in archives of many different convents" but he did not find a single case. However, Gagnon admitted that 1500 files were destroyed and another 2000 "could not be verified". He was "stupefied, not to say alarmed" by this negative finding and embarked on another search, this time using records from several pathological laboratories. In this search he identified three cases of cervical cancer in nuns. He concluded that "it was necessary, in my opinion, that very exceptionally at least this variety of cancer be found in virgin women".

Janet Towne, in a somewhat more reliable study, often misquoted as supporting Gagnon, stated that her own results were "quite different from those of Gagnon, in that 6 virginal women were recorded with proved cervical carcinoma, 3 having occurred in our own series of cases and 3 from the general survey" [6].

There is an interesting, rarely quoted, study from Holland, based on the Registrar-General's vital statistics from the period 1931-35: cervical cancer in nuns accounted for 2.5% of all cancer deaths in nuns (5/197), which was about the same as for wives of university teachers (2/70) and even higher than in farmers' wives (20/1183) [7].

In a survey of mortality in German nuns, Schömig found that cancer in nuns and in the general (female?) population was equally frequent (13.2 vs 13.4%, respectively) [8]. The nuns had a life expectancy about 10 years less than the general population. The frequency of genital carcinoma in nuns and in the general population was the same (23.6 vs 24.7% of all cancers, respectively). Of seven genital cancers in nuns, for which the site was specified, one was cervical cancer, four were cancers of the corpus, and two were ovarian cancers.

In a recent study on the mortality of nuns in Britain, Kinlen found 20 deaths from carcinoma of the uterus (site unspecified) against 28 expected. After 1941, when cervical cancer became to be classified separately, two nuns died of cervical cancer against 10 expected [9]. In a survey of three orders of nuns in the U.S.A., Taylor *et al* found, in a cohort born between 1870 and 1889, eight carcinomas of the uterus against an expected figure of 18 [10].

Fraumeni *et al.* collected 5893 death certificates among 41 religious orders. "Only white, native-born, never-married sisters" were included, while those who "had performed household or manual duties, were nurses, or had served at foreign missions" were excluded. Among 1021 cancer deaths there were 102 uterine cancers (76 site unspecified, 15 cancers of the corpus, 11 cancers of the cervix) [11].

Prostitutes, venereal disease, and cervical cancer
The paucity of good data on cervical cancer in prostitutes is even more striking than in nuns. The nineteenth-century doctors thought that uterine cancer was rare in prostitutes. Thus, for example, Drysdale wrote: "The evidence of Duchalet, Acton, Lippert, Bare of Nantes, and others, show incontestably that the health of prostitutes is above that of women in general. The only two diseases which infect them peculiarly being syphilis and scabies. Cancer of the womb is rare among prostitutes. Lippert of Hamburgh had not seen a case in eleven years among them" [12]. The best study is over 30 years old: Røjel found among 1262 patients with cervical cancer attending the Radium Centre in Copenhagen, 40 prostitutes (3.2%) and he calculated that prostitutes were four times more likely to be among the cases than among the controls [13]. All Røjel's prostitutes belonged to the lowest socioeconomic stratum, but the data were not corrected for this.

Other studies are summarised in Table 1 [14-27]. Only two studies deal specifically with prostitutes [19,22], though it was implied or stated in other studies, particularly those of prison populations, that a part of the clientele were prostitutes. The studies provide no evidence that cervical cancer is a more common cause of death in prostitutes than in other women. The Taiwan study explicitly contradicted the belief that "prostitution predisposes to increased rates of cervical cancer" [22]. The term "carcinoma in situ" (CIS) in these studies was used promiscuously, without histological definition and verification, and occasionally meant nothing more than a "positive smear"; yet, in the titles of these studies the term was shortened simply to "cancer". In one study, in which one third of the prisoners were alleged to be indulging in "prolonged scortatory* practices", the only case of invasive carcinoma occurred in a woman not classified as a prostitute [15].

The lack of relationship between venereal disease and cervical cancer was discussed by Gardner and Lyon [28]. However, I have included data on the prevalence of "carcinoma in situ" in patients attending VD clinics, together with some early and more recent prevalence studies on "carcinoma in situ" in various populations, for comparison (see Table 1). While none of these data are reliable and do not reflect the true incidence of either "premalignant" lesions or of invasive carcinoma, their wide scatter casts doubt on the interpretation of uncontrolled studies used as evidence that cervical cancer is "common" in prostitutes.

Lessons for health education

The link between cervical cancer and prostitution, *pace* the experts' opinion, is not " well documented". Statements such as "if one were to grade women by their sexual experience, from virgin to prostitute, the incidence of cervical cancer would be related to the amount of sexual exposure" [29] are sexist and degrading. Similarly, the term "promiscuity", often used in the literature on cervical cancer, is unhelpful. According to some authors, "promiscuity" means "sexual intercourse with more than one partner" [30] or with more than two [31]. It seems that promiscuity, if it means anything, is having more sex than the investigator. In a Dutch study on cervical cancer, 83% of cases had only one partner, and after controlling for the age at first coitus, the number of partners had no separate effect on the relative risk of

---

*The word "scortatory" is not in English dictionaries, but appears to be derived from the Latin *scortor* (to whore), *scortum* (a concubine).

invasive carcinoma in screened vs unscreened women [32].

Epidemiological research cannot prove causation. Observations which may have a bearing on hypotheses about the aetiology of cervical cancer should not be used for imputing causation and for blaming the

Table 1

Type of population	N	Prevalence of "carcinoma in situ" (per 1000) (CIS)	Prevalence of invasive cancer (per 1000)	Ref
VD clinic (Arkansas) poor blacks	3,224	12	9	14
Prison (California)	601	23	2	15
VD clinic (London)	235	9	9	16
VD clinic (Washington)	1,849	5	1	17
VD clinic (Birmingham)	1,500	11	0	18
Prison (London) prostitutes	185	86	0	19
Prison (Detroit)	460	39*	0	20
Prison (Montreal)	337	18†	12	21
Prostitutes (Taiwan)	750	11‡	0	22
Population screening (Tennessee) blacks	29,372	31	28	23
whites	53,585	23	19	
"Indigent" screening (Florida)	1,039	30	3	24
General practice screening (Derby)	807	14	1	25
Antenatal clinic (Brighton)	2,586	10	0	26
Population screening (Scotland)	18,321	8	?	27

*Compared to the prevalence of "CIS" in a planned-parenthood group (11/1000) and "indigent" prenatal patients (15/1000).
†compared to the prevalence of "CIS" in employees of Bell Telephone Co. (5/1000).
‡"Dysplasia plus".

victim. It is also dangerous to use the results of case-control studies as a basis for mass intervention measures. For example, when it was believed that the cause of cervical cancer was smegma ("proved" experimentally by inserting equine smegma into murine vaginas), the editor of the JAMA called for circumcision of all infants of poor parents, as it would be "more practical and thorough" than to teach the proletariat "good penile hygiene" [33]. Similarly, when the health educators convinced themselves that cervical cancer was directly related to a high frequency of coitus, a Senior Medical Officer from the British Department of Health announced that "the time was ripe for a campaign"; in the same breath he warned against "a very real danger... in fostering the idea that [cervical] cancer... may be associated with venereal disease" [34]. A few years later, it is now argued by some epidemiologists that cervical cancer is not only "associated" with venereal disease but that it is a venereal disease. Only a minority still resists the notion: "although this is called a venereal disease and the press have associated it with promiscuity, in fact the greatest risk factor ... is that of age and related to all sexually active women" [35]. It is uncharitable to accuse the Press of spreading false rumours, when the Press lifted their story directly from the epidemiological literature. And if a question of priority for the claim that cervical cancer is a venereal disease should ever arise, then Jean Astruc, an eighteenth-century French physician, should be considered, as he included among the causes of uterine cancer "injection of semen tainted with lues" and "venereal virus" [36].

The link between cervical cancer and misbehaviour preoccupies some experts: one epidemiologist showed that patients with cervical cancer were seven times more likely to have first coitus on the ground than in bed, and he provided details of the relative risks for 22 different ways of masturbating [37].

It is not helpful to argue with an assumption which remains to be proved. It begs the question. In one study, three women with cervical cancer said that they had only one partner: the investigators, believing in the promiscuity theory, disbelieved their informants: "the most likely explanation is that either husband or wife had in fact more than one sexual partner" [38]. The widespread decline in the incidence and mortality of cervical cancer in developed countries in the last 50 years has been interpreted as due to "less recourse to prostitutes than the older generation" [39]. It would be equally logical to argue that the decline was due to a general increase in chastity [40].

If cervical cancer were a venereal disease, the consequences might include: (1) screening and treating (?) healthy male carriers; this could be made compulsory before entering into a marriage contract; (2) screening for other venereal diseases at the time of the cervical smear; (3) exclusion from screening programmes of monogamous women, provided that their husband is "negative", as "strictly monogamous couples ... have negligible risk" [38]; the end of mass screening programmes, since only women with a "promiscuous" past, or married to "promiscuous" husbands who do not use condoms, would be at risk; (5) a positive smear would be a smear on the woman's character; (6) resurrection of the popular belief, fought against by health educators for decades, that cancer is an infectious, transmissible disease.

Before all this happens, more work perhaps should be done on unresolved issues, such as (i) the aetiology of cervical cancer, and (ii) the role of viruses, if any, in the aetiology. It is also important that cases of carcinoma of the cervix in virgins are carefully documented; it seems that gynaecologists are aware of such cases but they may be inhibited from publishing them, fearing that they would not be believed. One of the reviewers of this paper stated that "there is no question that cervical cancer can and does occur in women who have not been engaged in sexual activity". This opinion is in a startling contrast with views of others, e.g. Maisin's: "the nuns and the women who remain virgins never develop cervical cancer" [41].

Lest this communication be misrepresented, I wish to make it clear that I do not intend to imply that cervical cancer is in no way related to what the old gynaecologists (such as Gagnon) used to call "cervicitis" — an ill-defined term encompassing some normal conditions and also lesions due to infectious, chemical, and other agents. Mine is a moral tale and not a contribution to the enigma of the aetiology of cervical cancer. Some authors still believe firmly in herpes simplex virus type 2 (HSV-2) as a causative factor in cervical cancer; they are now in the minority. As pointed out in a recent authoritative review: "the most informative prospective investigation revealed no relationship between HSV-2 and subsequent cervical neoplasia" [42]. Similarly, a recent Lancet editorial stated that "the strong association between sexual activity and cervical cancer has encouraged the search for a sexually transmissible agent that could initiate or promote cervical neoplasia. Spirochaetes, spermatozoa, smegma, *Trichomonas vaginalis*, *Chlamydia trachomatis*, and HSV-2 have all come under suspicion, but proof of carcinogenesis has been lacking in every case" [43].

The latest of the putative venereal culprits is a human papilloma virus. It is however by no means clear that its only mode of transmission is a sexual contact: about 40% of normal oral biopsies in one study showed the presence of HPV-16 DNA, i.e. the type believed to be causally associated with cervical carcinoma [44]. HPV-16 has been found as often in cervical biopsies in normal women as in women with cervical cancer, if age-adjustment was carried out [45]. The presence of HPV-16 in cervical tissue does not correlate with lesions clinically diagnosed as CIN [46]. The frequency of HPV infection in the cervix decreases with age, while the frequency of invasive carcinoma increases with age [47]. As the Lancet editorialist concluded: "the high prevalence of papilloma-virus infection in women with cytologically and colposcopically normal cervices casts further doubts on the oncogenic role of these viruses" [43].

Conclusion

The epidemiological evidence on the prevalence of cervical cancer in nuns and prostitutes is of very poor quality and neither supports nor contradicts the belief that cervical cancer is a venereal disease. The evidence is so poor that it should not be used as additional "evidence" for a hypothesis which remains to be proved. Failure to distinguish hypotheses from facts delays clarification of the problem of the aetiology of cervical cancer.

References

1. Drife JO. *Br Med J* 1984; 288: 992.
2. Rotkin ID. Relation of adolescent coitus to cervical cancer risk. *JAMA* 1962; 179: 386-491.
3. Cislaghi C. Rilettura delle note del dott. Rigoni-Stern sulla frequenza del cancro, Verona 1842. *Epidemiol Prevenzione* 1978; No 3: 48-54.
4. [Rigoni-Stern]. Fatti statistici relativi alle malattie cancerose che servirono di base alle poche cose dette dal dott. Rigoni-Stern il di 23 settembre alla Sottosezione di chirurgia del IV Congresso degli scienzati Italiani. *Giornale per Servire ai Progressi della Patologia e della Terapeutica (Venezia)* 2 1842; (2nd series): 507-517.
5. Gagnon F. Contribution to the study of the etiology and prevention of cancer of the cervix of the uterus.
   Am J Obstet Gynecol 1950; 60: 516-522.
6. Towne JE. Carcinoma of the cervix in nulliparous and celibate women. *Am J Obstet Gynecol* 1955; 69: 606-613.
7. Versluys JJ. Cancer and occupation in the Netherlands.
   Br J Cancer 1949; 3: 161-185.
8. Schömig G. Die weiblichen Genitalkarzinome bei sexueller Enthaltsamkeit. *Strahlentherapie* 1953; 92: 156-158.
9. Kinlen LJ. Meat and fat consumption and cancer mortality: a study of strict religious orders in Britain. *Lancet* 1982; i: 946-949.
10. Taylor RS, Carroll BE, Lloyd JW. Mortality among women in three Catholic religious orders with special reference to cancer. *Cancer* 1959; 12: 1207-1225.
11. Fraumeni JF, Lloyd JW, Smith EM, Wagoner JK. Cancer mortality among nuns: role of marital status in etiology of neoplastic disease in women. *J Natl Cancer Inst* 1969; 42: 455-468.
12. Drysdale C. On the medical aspects of prostitution.
    Med Press 1866; i: 123-125.
13. Røjel J. The Interrelation between Uterine Cancer and Syphilis. A Patho-Demographic Study. A Busck, Copenhagen, 1953.
14. Nelson RB, Hilberg AW. The diagnosis of unsuspected cancer of the cervix. *J Natl Cancer Inst* 1951; 11: 1081-1089.

15. Pereyra AJ. The relationship of sexual activity to cervical cancer. Cancer of the cervix in a prison population. *Obstet Gynecol* 1961; 17: 154-159.
16. Farrer CJ. Tatham PH. Screening for carcinoma of the uterine cervix in a VD clinic. *Br J Vener Dis* 1962; 38: 230-231.
17. Pedersen AHB. Cytological screening for cancer in a venereal disease program. *Public Health Rep* 1964; 79: 1112-1118.
18. Lucas AJ, Williams DR. Cervical cytology of patients attending a venereal disease clinic. *J Obstet Gynaecol Br Commonwealth* 1967; 74: 104-110.
19. Keighley E. Carcinoma of the cervix among prostitutes in a women's prison. *Br J Vener Dis* 1968; 44: 254-255.
20. Moghissi KS, Mack HC, Porzak JP. Epidemiology of cervical cancer: study of a prison population. *Am J Obstet Gynecol* 1968; 100: 607-614.
21. Audet-Lapointe P. Detection of cervical cancer in a women's prison. *Can Med Assoc J* 1971; 104: 509—511.
22. Sebastian JA, Leeb BO. See R. Cancer of the cervix- a sexually transmitted disease. Cytological screening in a prostitute population. *Am J Obstet Gynecol* 1978; 131: 620-623.
23. Dunn JE. Preliminary findings of the Memphis-Shelby County uterine cancer study and their interpretation. *Am J Public Health* 1958; 48: 861-873.
24. Fulghum JE, Klein RJ. Community cancer demonstration project in Dade County., Florida. *Public Health Rep* 1962; 77: 165-170.
25. Lawrence RAAR. Exfoliative cytology in the early detection of cervical carcinoma in general practice. *J R Coll Gen Pract* 1968; 16: 379-391.
26. Andrews FJ, Linehan JJ, Melcher DH. Cervical cancer in younger women. *Lancet* 1978; ii: 776-778.
27. Duguid HLD, Duncan ID, Currie J. Screening for cervical intra-epithelial neoplasia in Dundee and Angus, 1962-81, and its relation with invasive cervical cancer. *Lancet* 1985; ii: 1053-1056.
28. Gardner JW, Lyon JL. Cancer of the cervix: a sexually transmitted infection? *Lancet* 1974; ii: 470-471.
29. Shimkin MB. New dimensions in cancer research. *Public Health Rep* 1963; 78: 195-206.

30. Beirão de Almeida A, Callegari TR. Relationship between the age of the beginning of the sexual activity and socio-economic status in the incidence of carcinoma of the uterine cervix. In: Nieburgs HE, ed. Prevention and Detection of Cancer. M Dekker; New York, 1978: 65-74.
31. Zaninetti P, Franseschi S, Baccolo M, Bonazzi B, Gottardi G, Serraion D. Characteristics of women under 20 with cervical intraepithelial neoplasia. *Int J Epidemiol* 1986; 15: 477-482.
32. Graaf van der Y, Zielhuis A, Peer PGM, Vooijs PG. The effectiveness of cervical screening: a population-based case-control study. *J Clin Epidemiol* 1988; 41: 21-26.
33. Anon. Epidemiology of cancer of the cervix. (Editorial). *JAMA* 1960; 174: 1852-1853.
34. Adams MJT. The prevention of cancer. *Ann R Coll Surg Engl* 1967; 41: 152-159.
35. Husain OAN. In discussion to Singer A, French P. Natural history and epidemiology of cervical carcinoma. In: McBrien DCH, Slater TF, eds. Cancer of the Uterine Cervix. Academic Press, London, 1984: 30.
36. Astruc J. A Treatise on all Diseases incident to Women. (Translated by J R...n.) Cooper; London, 1743: 220.
37. Rotkin ID. Sexual characteristics of a cervical cancer population. *Am J Public Health* 1967; 57: 815-829.
38. Buckley JD, Harris RWC, Doll R, Vessey MP, Williams PT. Case-control study of the husbands of women with dysplasia or carcinoma of the cervix uteri. *Lancet* 1981; ii: 1010-1015.
39. Skegg DCG, Corwin PA, Paul C, Doll R. Importance of the male factor in cancer of the cervix. *Lancet* 1982; ii: 581-583.
40. Skrabanek P, Jamieson M. Eaten by worms: a comment on cervical screening. *NZ Med J* 1985; 98: 654.
41. Maisin H, Vandenbroucke-Vanderwielen A, Sergent-Millet MA. Merckt van de J. Evaluation of high-risk groups of breast and cervix cancers in mass screening. In: Nieburgs HE, ed. Prevention and Detection of Cancer, Part 1. Dekker. New York, 1978: 2119-2134.
42. Brinton LA, Fraumeni JF. Epidemiology of uterine cervical cancer. *J Chron Dis* 1986; 39: 1051-1065.

43. Anon. Human papillomaviruses and cervical cancer: a fresh look at the evidence. (Editorial). *Lancet* 1987; i: 725-726.
44. Maitland NJ, Cox MF, Lynas C, Prime SS, Meanwell CA, Scully C. Detection of human papillomavirus DNA in biopsies of human oral tissue. *Br J Cancer* 1987; 56: 245-250.
45. Meanwell CA, Cox MF, Blackledge G, Maitland NJ. HPV 16 DNA in normal and malignant cervical epithelium: implications for the aetiology and behaviour of cervical neoplasia. *Lancet* 1987; i: 703-707.
46. Murdoch JB, Cordiner JW, Macnab JCM. Relevance of HPV 16 to laser therapy for cervical lesions. *Lancet* 1987; i: 1433.
47. De Villiers E-M, Wagner D, Schneider A, Wesch H, Miklaw H, Wahrendorf J, Papendick U, zur Hausen H. Human papillomavirus in women with and without abnormal cervical cytology. *Lancet* 1987; ii: 703-706.

8

IS ANIMAL EXPERIMENTATION STILL NECESSARY?

Progress in life sciences would be unthinkable without experiments using live animals and animal tissues. Of 71 Nobel Prizes for Physiology and Medicine, 63 were awarded to scientists for discoveries based on animal experimentation (Ullrich and Creutzfeldt, 1985).

The rhetorical question in the title of this section can be answered 'no' only if the corollary question, 'Is progress in life sciences still necessary?' is also answered with 'no'. This is the hub of the matter. Those who are opposed to progress in medicine and science are the lucky people who did not have a painful, incurable disease, or who do not have to nurse their own dying child.

Science, of which life sciences are a part, is not pursued with the sole aim of reducing human suffering; searching for knowledge is a human attribute, inseparable from man, just as speech, art or humour. Science is often criticised for being immoral. Henri Poincaré, whom Bertrand Russell called the most eminent scientist of his generation, wrote that science and ethics can never be in conflict because the domain of science (search for knowledge) and the domain of ethics (search for norms of conduct) only touch each other, but they do not overlap. In other words, science cannot be immoral, though some scientists pursue knowledge by immoral means, and, conversely, ethics cannot be scientific, although some moralists make absolute claims. Science chooses which goal to pursue, which horizon to push further, while ethics tell us by which means we are allowed to achieve it (Poincaré, 1904).

Ethical rules are meaningful only when the majority of people accept them as reasonable and agree to enforce them. It is silly to speak about 'animal rights' in a society which uses animals for food, clothing and sport. What is 'animal' anyway? Man is an animal. A fly is an animal.

What rights should blue-bottles be allocated? Or should only cuddly mammals have rights? Should voles have the right not to be eaten by the fox, and mice the right not to be slowly killed by the cat? We live in an era of 'rights' at a time when the majority of mankind is denied the basic needs for a decent life. The emptiness of the language of rights was seen long ago by Jeremy Bentham who said that to speak about rights is nonsense, and to speak about natural rights is a nonsense upon stilts.

The increased public interest in the 'anti-vivisectionist' movement, together with the birth of a new branch of ethics which deals with the 'animal rights', is due to a variety of factors, some of them based on genuine fear and concern about the direction science is taking, while the others represent the dark, obscurantist streaks of anti-intellectualism opposing progress throughout human history. These two main strands, interwoven in the anti-vivisection propaganda, must first be disentangled.

Some experiments on animals are not necessary and are therefore indefensible. However, for a less informed member of the public, it may be difficult to decide what is necessary and what is not. For example, when the famous neuro-physiologist Brown-Séquard was given a sharp blow across the fingers with an umbrella by a lady who was present at one of his demonstrations, in which he was using a monkey, at the Collège de France in 1883, the lady did not know that Brown-Séquard's experiments enormously advanced our understanding of the function of the nervous system and the spinal cord. And how many more experiments will be necessary before we can offer hope to some paralysed victims (Anon, 1883).

Not all experiments on animals serve science, e.g. toxicity testing and safety control for substances used or consumed by humans. When such testing involves new cosmetics, lipsticks etc., it is not enough to have calls for the abolition of such tests from people who do not use such products themselves. Society must be informed about the nature of the tests and then decide whether they want more cosmetics or not.

Some animal experiments represent a useless repetition for the sake of producing 'research' papers which will be used by the author for filling the space under 'Publications' in an application for a better job. This can be prevented by establishing the competence of the researcher, by assessing the objectives of the proposed animal experiments, and by supervision. The mechanisms for this exist. For example, in England, inspectors from the Home Office, which is responsible for supervising adherence to the regulations about animal experimentation, made on average, 13 surprise visits a year to each registered centre for animal experimentation. This compares very favourably with the frequency of inspections of factories where considerable human hazard exists — about one a year (Paton, 1984).

While some animal experiments are unnecessary, the scientists would be the first to admit that much of the activity which passes under the name 'science' is not worthy of its name. Scientific literature is replete with peer criticism of slipshod research. Where animals (or humans) are used for unjustified, poorly planned experiments, such practices should be exposed, criticised and their repetition prevented.

A more complicated problem is the use of animals (or humans) for research in behavioural control. There is a potential gain in better understanding of the causes and treatment of mental diseases, although the use of animals as models of human mental disease appears to me absurd (Skrabanek, 1984). However, some of this research has been sponsored, directly or indirectly, by the military, and the implications are obvious: the results could be useful in controlling the minds of healthy people who are classified as 'enemies'. The public, and conscientious scientists, are rightly concerned about this type of research; and its nature and value should be scrutinised in informed debate.

Experiments which induce suffering and pain are also an area of contention. Proper use of anaesthesia answers some, but not all the objections. However, the anti-vivisectionists tend to forget that many diseases, whose causes and treatment the scientists try to discover by animal experimentation, also causes pain and suffering to human victims and their families. To avoid all suffering is impossible. The human lot is a tragic one, and will remain so, if the human race does not terminate the tragedy by annihilating itself.

While conceding all reasonable objections to unnecessary animal experimentation and to inflicting unjustifiable pain on animals, I would now like to turn to the second main trend in the anti-vivisectionist movement—the opposition to science; the opposition to the advancement of knowledge.

Since Adam was expelled from Paradise, we know that we cannot spit out the apple with the 'worm' of knowledge and revert to the state of blissful ignorance. Since Prometheus stole fire from the gods, we know that we cannot put the gifts of Pandora back into her amphora. Rousseau's call to go back to nature, so dear to present-day utopians, appeals only to those who prefer wishful thinking to the harsh reality of the human predicament. The apostles of anti-science, such as Theodore Roszak, want us 'to ground science in a sensibility drawing on the occult, mysticism, the Romantic movement...' (Wade, 1972).

Nature is mysterious and will remain so. For a scientist there is only one way: to stumble forward in the darkness without turning back. For anti-scientists, this would be a nightmare; they have a horror of not knowing, they have to deny ignorance by filling in the blank with wishful fantasy. As Erasmus observed, 'man's mind is so formed that it is far more susceptible to falsehood than to truth .... The fools are better off, first because their happiness costs them so little, in fact only a grain of persuasion, secondly because they share their enjoyment of it with the majority of men (Erasmus, 1512).

Acupuncturists do not have to do any animal experiments. They know it all. They understand the causes and treatments of all diseases. So do the practitioners of other 'alternative' medicines. But alternative medicine is no alternative. Roszak ridicules the objective knowledge of science: he and his ilk wish us to return to alchemy, astrology and irrational subjectivism. This is an ostrich-like attitude to human suffering. The 18th century English physician, Thomas Beddoes, put the following words under the heading 'Experiments in medicine' in his notebook: "Those who decry them do not perhaps perceive that they cut off all hope from those at present incurable".

It is often alleged that animal experimentation in medical school is a deliberate attempt to desensitise future doctors. Surely they are more effectively desensitised by encountering their first 'patient' as a pickled cadaver. In fact, some desensitization is desirable: should a doctor faint when he sees his patient bleeding?

Compassion for humans is not necessarily accompanied by pity for humans. As pointed out by a *Lancet* correspondent, had the millions of human victims of Nazi-occupied Europe qualified under the laws protecting animals, as introduced by H. Goering, their fate might have been different (Seidelman, 1986). Some modern anti-vivisectionists would still prefer experiments on live humans than dead animals. This reminds me of a French surgeon who taught Western medicine in China and asked for some corpses which he could use for dissection. This request was received with horror by his Chinese employees, who nevertheless, assured the surgeon that he could have an unlimited supply of live criminals (Russell, 1950).

Recently, the Greater London Council allowed the British Union for the Abolition of Vivisection and the National Anti-Vivisection Society to erect a statue in a public park to a dog, which in 1903 (according to the inscription) "endured vivisections—till death came to his release" (Anon, 1985). The inscription did not mention that the dog was operated upon (always with anaesthesia) by E.H. Starling, W.M. Bayliss and Henry Dale, most brilliant British scientists, and that the experiments led to the discovery of the first hormone and to the birth of modern endocrinology.

The most powerful argument of the anti-vivisectionist extremists, who campaign for abolition of all animal experiments without exception, is presented in books by Hans Ruesch. I own the American version (Ruesch, 1983). It is a *j'accuse* type of book, in which no hold is barred if it serves the Cause. It is a book which makes converts readily, including medical doctors. (This is not surprising since doctors have to endure dogmatic education which discourages critical thinking.)

Is animal experimentation still necessary?

Much of what Mr. Ruesch says is true, but it is half-truths which he exploits with great effect. He accuses scientists of "greed, cruelty, ambition, incompetence, vanity, callousness, stupidity, sadism and insanity". I have seen it myself, but which category of people is immune to these charges, including writers to which Mr. Ruesch belongs? Mr. Ruesch finds it hilarious that studies of the 'love life of the flea' and of 'the mating call of the mosquito' attract funding. Is he not aware that the fleas are the vectors of the plague, and the mosquitoes of malaria? Better understanding of their reproduction could save millions of human lives. Some of Mr. Ruesch's accusations are malicious: "insulin treatment has done more damage than it brought benefits, has killed more people than it has saved". He has to say this, since insulin was discovered by animal experimentation, therefore such a discovery must be a Pyrrhic victory for scientists. Mr. Reusch's alternatives are bizarre: 'medical science today knows nothing with certainty that Hippocrates didn't know already'. He does not say that Hippocrates' humours (blood, phlegm, yellow bile and black bile) have now only humorous value. Not surprisingly, Mr. Ruesch approves and recommends homeopathy, osteopathy and acupuncture: 'they raise medical art gradually up to the Hippocratic level again'.

Fortunately, not all animal welfare groups hold such extreme views, and most of them have an important role to play in finding the proper balance between animal welfare and human needs. In Great Britain, the Cruelty to Animals Act of 1876 has become inadequate for regulating animal experimentation, and a new version, known as the Animals (Scientific Experimentation) Bill is now being debated in the House of Commons. The British Veterinary Association, the Committee for the Reform of Animal Experimentation, and the Fund for the Replacement of Animals in Medical Experiments have welcomed the Bill. As these organizations jointly stated, what we need is an effective compromise between the welfare of animals, the legitimate demands of the public for accountability and the equally legitimate requirements of medicine, science and commerce. In a reasonable society a reasonable compromise must be found.

References

Anon. *J Am Med Assoc* 1883; 1: 28.

Anon. A new anti-vivisectionist libellous statue at Battersea. *Br Med J* 1986; 292: 683.

Erasmus of Rotterdam (1512). In praise of folly. Translated by B. Radice. Penguin Books, Harmondsworth, 1971.

Paton W. Man and Mouse. Oxford University Press, Oxford, 1984.

Poincaré H. . La Valeur de la Science. Flammarion, Paris. 1904.

Ruesch H. Slaughter of the Innocent. Civitas Publications, New York, 1983.

Russell B. An outline of intellectual rubbish. In: Unpopular Essays. Allen and Unwin, London, 1950.

Seidelman WE. Animal experiments in Nazi Germany. *Lancet* 1986; i: 1214.

Stock JE. Memoirs of the life of Thomas Beddoes. John Murray, London, 1811.

Skrabanek P. Biochemistry of schizophrenia: a pseudo-scientific model. *Integrative Psychiatry* 1984; 2: 224.

Ullrich KJ. and Creutzfeldt OD. Gesundheit und Tierschutz. ECON Verlag, Düsseldorf and Wien, 1985.

Wade N. (1972). Theodore Roszak: visionary critic of science. *Science* 178, 960.

9

NONSENSUS CONSENSUS

When in 1974 the American Psychiatric Association declared that homosexuality was no longer a disease, the new consensus was the result of a vote among the members. Similarly, if a group of religious functionaries were to cast a vote on whether homosexuality is still a sin, the majority could give their assent and the consensus would be upheld. It would be a mistake to equate such consensuses with a democratic decision, as *demos* has no say in the matters. Neither is anyone the wiser when a consensus is reached.

Consensus conferences on health issues are a recent phenomenon. Since 1977, the National Institutes of Health in the USA have organised almost 100 consensus conferences, at a cost of about $10 million. Most doctors are unaware of what these conferences were about and in many instances the practice of medicine has been unaffected. As recommendations from consensus conclaves are issued *ex cathedra*, without any reference to original data, lawyers may use them in malpractice suits against doctors who have not followed them. The careful selection of participants guarantees a consensus. A token dissident, coopted to maintain the semblance of impartiality, is, as a rule, not given space to ruffle the smoothness of the consensus report. Yet the very need for consensus stems from a lack of consensus. Why make an issue of agreeing on something that everyone (or nearly everyone) takes for granted? In science, lack of consensus does not bring about the urge to hammer out a consensus by assembling participants whose dogmatic views are well known and who welcome an opportunity to have them reinforced by mutual backslapping. On the contrary, scientists

---

This paper first appeared with the title 'Viewpoint: Nonsensus consensus' in *The Lancet* 1990; 335: 1446-1447. © The Lancet Ltd. Reproduced by kind permission of The Lancet Ltd.

are provided with a strong impetus to go back to the benches and do more experiments.

Uncertainty in medicine, as in theology, is intolerable and a consensus conference, like a synod of bishops, is convoked to settle the matter. A recent example was the report of the National Cholesterol Education Program Expert Panel on detection, evaluation and treatment of high blood cholesterol, issued by a committee of thirty experts.[1] There is strength in numbers and it silences the critics. Among many recommendations, this report endorses a diet for which there is not a scrap of evidence that it is capable of changing the risk of dying from coronary heart disease, but there is reasonable evidence that it does not. The agreement on dietary treatment and on the meaning of "high" cholesterol is achieved by an old Chinese consensus method employed in settling the question of the length of the Emperor's nose. As Richard Feynman recalled, since no one was allowed to see the Emperor's face, this precluded direct measurement, but a consensus could still be reached by going around the kingdom and asking experts on the length of the Emperor's nose what they *thought* it might be and by averaging all the answers. Since the number of questioned imperial rhinosophists was rather large, the standard error of the mean was very low, and the precision of the estimate was good.

Medical fashions come and go, but now that the world has become a global village, they reap hecatombs of victims. People have developed a new love-hate relationship with medicine: they dream about "alternatives" but they pay through the nose for "health checks". The financial exploitation of the worried-well and of the sick whom doctors cannot cure is no longer verbally denounced by the leaders of the profession; it is the order of the day. To make it easier for "consumers" to opt for buying "health", the "product" is neatly packaged and advertised with slogans that have a scientific ring—computerised diagnosis, automated cholesterol measurement, the latest pharmaceutical breakthroughs, and other quick technological fixes for human ills and woes. The risks of new technologies are not evaluated; and since there is no evidence of risks it is assumed that there is evidence of no risks. When finally the risks can no longer be ignored and exceed the benefits by a wide margin, a new fashion takes over. It took over ten years for neonatologists to question why over 10,000 premature babies in incubators became blind. The cause of the blindness was retrolental fibroplasia induced by the use of oxygen. The possibility that something so good and natural as oxygen could become a leading cause of childhood blindness did not cross anyone's mind for a long time. It is easy to be wise with hindsight. But what about the "prudent" diet, recommended by experts who claim that if ingested daily it would conquer the number one killer—coronary heart disease? Surely it could do no harm, or could it?

Consensus experts do not put any cost on their recommendations since everyone would live longer and who are we to put a price on human life? Money spent on one crusade will not be available for other, more effective uses. For this very reason it would be unwise for a single-cause enthusiast to delve too deeply: other experts could cheat him out of his budget. To make their case, the consensus experts are tempted to inflate the importance of their cause by jumbo-jet statistics. This is done by enumerating how many lives would be lost, which otherwise would be saved if the experts got hold of the money, in the next 10, 20, 50 years, in a population of 100, 200, 500 million. As such numbers are large, and become larger by multiplication, they can be expressed suitably as the number of jumbo jets crashing in the national airspace daily. These statistical massacres stun both politicians and the public. Once the bandwagon starts moving downhill the prestige, power, and credibility of the expert are at stake. Various ruses must be employed to suppress, dismiss, or distort new information which undermines the premises of the consensus.

There have been too many "disasters of good intent" in the history of medicine and people should temper their faith in experts — particularly when they see them coming in droves — with their own informed scepticism. After all, it is the public who will carry the cost both physically and financially. William Silverman pointed out that the ultimate test of any medical innovation should be, Is life any sweeter?

"Criticism must come from sceptics in the community if we are to separate 'halfway' technical solutions from solid claims of improvement in general welfare".[2] Knowing that someone is eager to sell you a cholesterol number, and keep the proceeds of the lottery, could put off even the hardened gambler.

The oldest consensus among the vendors of health, and other traders along the valley of the shadow of death, was that people want to be deceived and should be pleased accordingly. In the past, mountebanks were distinguishable from their more respectable colleagues at least in appearance and manners, if not by the effectiveness of their cures. Nowadays, the convergence of medicine and its "alternatives" is an ominous foretaste of the ultimate consensus that all will be healthy by the year 2000, with the WHO blessing, provided they don't die by then, eat plenty of fibre, and promise never to use their reason again.

References

1. The Expert Panel. Report of the National Cholesterol Education Program on detection, evaluation, and treatment of high blood cholesterol in adults. *Arch Intern Med* 1988; 148: 36-69.
2. Silverman WA. Neonatal pediatrics at the century mark. *Persp Biol Med* 1989; 32: 159-70.

10

WHY IS PREVENTIVE MEDICINE EXEMPTED FROM ETHICAL CONSTRAINTS?

Author's abstract

It is a paradox that medical experimentation on individuals, whether patients or healthy volunteers, is now controlled by strict ethical guidelines, while no such protection exists for whole populations which are subjected to medical interventions in the name of preventive medicine or health promotion. As many such interventions are either of dubious benefit or of uncertain harm-benefit balance, such as mass screening for cancers or for risk factors associated with coronary heart disease, there is no justification for maintaining the ethical vacuum in which preventive medicine finds itself at present.

Ethics of human experimentation

History shows that the medical profession seldom puts its house in order unless under pressure from the public. It may not be generally appreciated that ethical guidelines governing human experimentation were never part of the medical code until public revulsion at scandalous experiments on human 'guinea-pigs' in the 1950s and 1960s which were sponsored by official medical bodies (1-5). Research ethics committees owe their existence to public concern, such as that which followed exposure of the Tuskegee experiment, conducted by the US Public Health Service and the Surgeon-General on some 400 poor blacks whose syphilis had been left untreated in order to study the natural progression of the disease. The patients' (if that is the word) co-operation was obtained by the promise of a free funeral. The study

---

This paper first appeared in the *Journal of Medical Ethics*, 1990, Volume 16, pages 187-190. Reproduced by kind permission of the BMJ Publishing Group.

was not stopped until 1972, not because the medical profession protested when they saw interim reports from this study in medical journals, but because a non-medical assistant leaked the details of the experiment to a reporter from the Associated Press (1). The subsequent Senate hearing resulted in the National Research Act, 1974, which contained specific provision for 'institutional review boards', that is ethical committees (6).

A more recent scandal, in 1989 in the United Kingdom, concerned unethical experimentation on over 30 patients with cancer, leukaemia or AIDS, in a private hospital in London, by a doctor who charged £ 10,000 for a course of unproved treatment (7). Again, it was an investigative journalist and television who brought this affair into the open (7).

Despite the nominal supervision of human experimentation by ethical committees, medical research on humans is often carried out in circumstances in which the patients are 'mostly passive participants, unwitting beneficiaries, or ignorant victims' (8). Herxheimer called for public involvement in the ethical issues of clinical trials (8). According to Tunkel, who is a barrister, a patient who takes part in a trial and suffers adverse effects has no legal right to compensation and should be informed beforehand accordingly (9).

There is no reason why this proper concern about the rights of patients in clinical trials to be fully informed about the nature of the experiment, its expected benefits and its potential harms should not be extended to population experiments conducted in the name of health promotion or preventive medicine.

The ethical vacuum of preventive medicine

At present, State or private bodies conducting mass preventive interventions have no obligation to inform the healthy participants that they are the subjects of experiments of uncertain outcome and potential harm. As the interventions are 'preventive medicine', they are automatically exempted from ethical constraints.

Why is preventive medicine exempted from ethical constraints ?

For example, in the Breast Cancer Detection Project set up in 1973 by the National Cancer Institute and the American Cancer Society to screen a quarter of a million healthy women, the possible risks of mammography were not explained to them nor were they told about the lack of evidence for the benefit of mammography in women under the age of fifty (10). In subsequent similar trials in different countries, no mention was made in the published reports whether the participants received adequate information about the uncertainties of benefit. Such information could, of course, jeopardise the 'compliance' rate and the 'throughput'.

The reasons for the ethical limbo in which preventive medicine finds itself are in part historical and in part political. Historically, preventive medicine grew out of the State's interest in protecting its productive, healthy citizens by the segregation of those who suffered contagious diseases such as leprosy or plague. Early preventive medicine was synonymous with medical policing. In the 19th century, prostitutes were screened by police surgeons not for the sake of their own health but for the protection of their clients. Screening for disease was initially used as a sieve to separate the healthy and useful from the weak and useless, whether on behalf of insurance companies (to exclude poor risks), armies (to weed out weaklings) or employers (to keep up productivity). In 1900, Lord Rosebery, an important political figure of the time, saw the problem of national health in terms of crude social Darwinism; in a speech at the University of Glasgow he stated: 'Where you promote health and arrest disease, where you convert an unhealthy citizen into a healthy one, where you exercise your authority to promote sanitary conditions and suppress those which are the reverse, you, in doing your duty are also working for the Empire ... Health of mind and body exalt a nation in the competition of the universe. The survival of the fittest is an absolute truth in the conditions of the modern world' (11).

Another reason why preventive medicine has so far been exempted from ethical considerations may be the half-truth that prevention is better than cure, with the implication that any possible disadvantage is more than repaid by the ensuing benefit. While this may be true for some preventive measures, such as immunisation or common-sense hygiene, it may not apply for other preventive activities, such as screening for cancer or for risk factors for coronary heart disease. Population interventions aimed at reducing coronary heart disease have been a spectacular failure (12), and, as regards cancer prevention, despite much military rhetoric and decades of expensive crusades, the war on cancer has been declared lost in at least one authoritative analysis (13). We should not confuse 'prevention' with 'hopes of prevention'. Uncovering problems for which there is no effective treatment is not preventive medicine but a medical contribution to ill-health.

Could preventive medicine be dangerous to health?

The proverb, 'a stitch in time saves nine', may be sound advice for mending socks but it makes little sense if a thousand people need one stitch (in its medical equivalent) to save one person from nine stitches. Translated into financial terms, 10 pence of prevention a day is not cheaper than £10 for a cure a year. Many preventive measures, such as cancer screening, require regular visits to the doctor or to a special clinic throughout life, may involve unpleasant or dangerous procedures, cause iatrogenic morbidity (and perhaps even death), and result in the medicalisation of life for all.

It is naively presumed that preventive medicine is a risk-free pursuit, which, at worst, may do no good. This is hardly a valid argument. As one wit observed, what would you say to a salesman who was offering you a new electric gimmick which failed to work on demonstration, when he beamed at you and said, 'but it didn't blow the fuse!'

Becker warned that health promotion 'fosters a dehumanising self-concern which substitutes personal health goals for more important, humane, societal goals. It is a new religion in which we worship ourselves, attribute good health to our devoutness, and view illness as just punishment for those who have not yet seen the Way' (14).

The harm of preventive medicine has been discussed and documented by various authors (15-18). Even something so innocuous as the adoption of a cholesterol-lowering diet, as prescribed by the American Heart Association, could increase rather than decrease the risk of coronary heart disease in women (19). The logical *non-sequitur* of lowering blood cholesterol in healthy people because cholesterol is a risk marker for coronary heart disease led to the tragedy of the clofibrate trial, in which significantly more healthy men treated with clofibrate died than the controls (12). It is unlikely that the men were informed beforehand about the possibility that their participation in the trial might be harmful to them and even fatal.

As up to 50 per cent of a population (depending on an arbitrary definition of 'elevated' cholesterol) is the potential target for mass intervention by preventionists (20), the pharmaceutical industry is eagerly anticipating the profits from the mountain of cholesterol-lowering medicaments which will be prescribed by doctors. Long-term effects of such treatment are not known but are unlikely to be harmless.

A similar situation exists in screening for hypertension. Hypertension is not a disease but an arbitrarily defined physical measure: not surprisingly, according to some 'experts', up to 40 per cent of adult populations are 'hypertensive'. The measurement of blood pressure in practice is uncertain and imprecise and consequently many people are labelled as 'hypertensive' on false grounds (21). The effects of such labelling are serious: they include the erosion of the sense of well-being, lowered sense of self-esteem, marital problems, reduction in earning power, and the adoption of a 'sick role' in a previously healthy person (22).

Women are particularly vulnerable to the exploits of preventive medicine. Great pressure is put on them to undergo regular gynaecological examinations, physical examinations of their breasts and to practise in addition breast self-examination. Some women doctors are starting to question the 'well-womanising' crusade, in which the major casualties are the women themselves (23).

Breast cancer screening has an adverse harm-benefit ratio, but women are told nothing about the nature and the extent of risks; these include unnecessary operations due to false-positive results, which far outnumber true-positive findings (24,25). Schmidt calculated that for each woman who benefits from screening, 18 women have to live longer with the knowledge of their incurable disease ('extra cancer years') because of earlier diagnosis by screening. This estimate was based on the best mammographical results, which have not been reproduced in other centres. Schmidt also pointed out, in his detailed critique of the Swedish mammographic trial, that over 100 women would have needle biopsy and further surgical investigations for each woman who could expect benefit in terms of a cure (26).

In cervical cancer screening, the possible benefits are debatable and may be non-existent, but the harms are common and largely ignored (27). The principal author of the British National Health Programme, Alwyn Smith, stated that 'it is absurd to conduct a screening test in such a way that nearly forty women are referred for an expensive and possibly hazardous procedure for every woman who is at risk of developing serious disease' (29). Yet this absurd situation continues unabated, without anyone recognising an obligation to the women to inform them about the true state of the 'art'.

Breast self-examination has never been shown to reduce mortality from breast cancer and there are theoretical reasons why it is unlikely to do so, because by the time breast cancer is palpable the tumour will have been growing for a long time. In the UK trial of early breast cancer detection this method was proved to be worthless (29), and it could be argued that it is actually harmful, particularly in younger women, as it leads to unnecessary anxiety and unnecessary medical and surgical intervention in the vast majority of women who discover an abnormality during the ritual of self-examination (30). Yet, as with other unproved preventive measures, cancer societies and other well-meaning but misguided groups are allowed freely to broadcast misleading propaganda. Breast cancer screening recommendations were described by one editorialist as 'a confusing mixture of half-truths, unsupported by the scientific evidence to date, which only adds to the anxiety and uncertainty that always seems to cloud rational discussion of what knowledge we do—or especially do not—have about breast cancer' (31).

Unfortunately, optimistic even though untrue information about prevention is more believable than sober, grim facts, and as such is readily exploited by medical profit-making organisations. In Ireland, 'executive health screening' is offered in a number of private clinics: charges range from £170 in the Charlemont Clinic to £200 in the Blackrock Clinic for men, while women who have in addition an optional cervical smear and mammography are charged £250 (32). BUPA in the UK run the following advertisement in the national papers: 'If you are almost positively certain that you're probably healthy, why not talk to BUPA? ... Health assessment costs £232 for men and £268 for women ... So don't kid yourself that you're healthy. Find out for sure by filling in the coupon below'.

In the absence of any ethical guidelines more and more unsuspecting people will be caught in the 'preventive' net.

In search of the ethics of preventive medicine

Population interventions which have as their goal the prevention of coronary heart disease and many cancers should be classified as population experiments and the same guidelines should apply to them as to clinical trials. That such interventions are of an experimental nature and of uncertain benefit is made clear by the fact that they are often tested in randomised controlled trials.

If a healthy volunteer, or a patient, has a right to be fully informed about the risks and benefits of the trial in which he takes part, even more meticulous attention should be paid to the rights of a whole population of healthy people who are subjected to mass prevention programmes and intervention, however well meant.

As Gillon pointed out, health education (and this applies equally to all areas of preventive medicine) is 'as heavily bedevilled by moral issues as is any other area of health care', and it should 'conform, as much as any other area of medical care, to the medico-moral norms of respect for people's autonomy, beneficence, non-maleficence, and justice' (33). In a penetrating analysis of the health-promotion industry, Williams noted that the field is riddled with serious conceptual and ethical problems, and expressed concern about the lack of protection of the public (by a medical equivalent of the Trades Description Act) against the hard-sell techniques of health salesmen (34).

A forum should be act up enabling representatives of the public, and of the medical and legal professions, to identify the ethical problems posed by new developments in preventive medicine and health promotion.

References

1 Jones JH. Bad blood. The Tuskegee syphilis experiment. The Free Press, New York, 1981.

2 US House of Representatives Subcommittee. American nuclear guinea pigs: three decades of radiation experiments on US citizens. US Goverment Printing Office, Washington, 1986.

3 Beecher HK. Ethical and clinical research. *New England Journal of Medicine* 1966; 274: 1354-1360.

4 Gillmor D. I swear by Apollo. Dr Ewen Cameron and the CIA-brainwashing experiments. Eden Press, Montreal, 1987.

5 Pappworth MH. Human guinea pigs. Experimentation on man. Penguin Books, Harmondsworth, 1969.

6 Capron A. Research ethics and the law. In: Berg K, Tranoy K E, eds. Research ethics. A Liss, New York, 1983: 17.

7 Anonymous. Scandal in Southwark. *Lancet* 1989; i: 856-857.

8 Herxheimer A. The rights of the patient in clinical research. *Lancet* 1988; ii: 1128-1130.

9 Tunkel V. Drug trials: who takes the risk? *Lancet* 1989; ii: 609-611.

10 Carbone PP. A lesson from the mammography issue.
Annals of internal medicine. 1978; 88: 703-704.

11 Eyler JM. Poverty, disease, responsibility: Arthur Newsholme and the public health dilemmas of British liberalism.
Millbank quarterly 1989; 67 (suppl 1): 109-129.

12 McCormick J, Skrabanek P. Coronary heart disease is not preventable by population interventions. *Lancet* 1988; ii: 839-841.

13 Bailer JC, Smith EM. Progress against cancer?
New England journal of medicine 1986; 314: 1226-1232.

14 Becker MH. The tyranny of health promotion.
Public health review 14:15-25.

15 Skrabanek P. Mass screening in women: more harm than benefit? In: Social dilemmas in cancer prevention. Macmillan Press, London, 1989: 67-73.

16 Marteau TM. Psychological costs of screening may sometimes be bad enough to undermine the benefits of screening.
British Medical Journal 1989; 299: 527

17 Stoate HG. Can health screening damage your health? *Journal of the Royal College of General Practitioners* 1989; 39: 193-195.

18 Tymstra T. False positive results in screening tests: experiences of parents of children screened for congenital hypothyroidism.
Family practice 1986; 3: 92-96.

19 Crouse JR. Gender, lipoproteins, diet, and cardiovascular risk. Sauce for the goose may not be sauce for the gander. *Lancet* 1989; i: 318-320.

20 Smith WCS, Kenicer MB, Davis AM, Evans AE, Yarnell J. Blood cholesterol: is population screening warranted in the UK? *Lancet* 1989; i: 372-373.

21 Anonymous. More on hypertensive labelling (editorial).
Lancet 1985; i: 1138-1139.

22 Alderman MH, Lamprot B. Labelling of hypertensives: a review of the data. *Journal of Clinical Epidemiology* 1990; 43: 195-200.

23 McCullogh S. Useless smear campaign.
    The Spectator 1989 Feb 11: 20-23.

24 Skrabanek P. The debate over mass mammography in Britain. The case against. *British Medical Journal* 1988; 297: 971-972.

25 Skrabanek P. Mass mammography: the time for reappraisal. *International journal of technology assessment in health care* 1989; 5: 423-430.

26 Schmidt JG. The epidemiology of mass breast cancer screening — a plea for a valid measure of benefit. *Journal of clinical epidemiology* 1990; 43: 215-225.

27 Skrabanek P. Cervical cancer screening: the time for reappraisal. *Canadian journal of public health* 1988; 79: 86-88.

28 Smith A. Cervical cytology screening. *British Medical Journal* 1988; 296: 1670.

29 UK trial of early detection of breast cancer group. First results on mortality reduction in the UK trial of early detection of breast cancer. *Lancet* 1989; ii: 411-416.

30 Frank JW, Mai V. Breast self-examination in young women: more harm than good? *Lancet* 1985; ii: 654-657.

31 Dixon T. Breast cancer: the debate continues. *Canadian family physician* 1987; 33: 817-818.

32 Anonymous. Health screening. Irish medical times (financial supplement) 1989 May.

33 Gillon R. Health education: the ambiguity of the medical role. In: Doxiadis S, ed. Ethics in health education. Wiley, Chichester, 1990: 29-41.

34 Williams G. Health promotion — caring concern or slick salesmanship? *Journal of medical ethics* 1994; 10: 191-195.

11

RISK-FACTOR EPIDEMIOLOGY: SCIENCE OR NON-SCIENCE?

The changing role of epidemiology

Until about 1950, epidemiologists studied patterns of infectious diseases, particularly the more common ones. The term *epidemia* was used since the time of Hippocrates for widespread diseases affecting whole populations (*epidemeo* to be among a people). As infectious diseases gradually became less prevalent, in part due to the discovery of antibiotics, epidemiologists had to turn their attention to something else. It is no longer clear what is the raison d'être of epidemiology, as judged for example from 23 different definitions of epidemiology, collected by Lilienfeld.[1] He points out that 'the idea that epidemiology is the study of anything is a very modern innovation'. In a sense, there is an epidemic of epidemiologists who are short of diseases suitable for their investigations.

The main preoccupation of epidemiologists is now the association game. This consists in searching for associations between 'diseases of civilisation' and 'risk factors'. The 'diseases of civilisation' are heart disease and cancer. The curse of civilisation is that people are deprived of dying young of simple infectious diseases, such as tuberculosis, smallpox, or the plague. The 'risk factors' studied by epidemiologists are either personal characteristics (age, sex, race, weight, height, diet, habits, customs, vices) or situational characteristics (geography, occupation, environment, air, water, sun, gross national product, stress, density of doctors).

This paper first appeared in Health, Lifestyle and Environment (D Anderson, Ed.), London; Social Affairs Unit; New York, Manhattan Institute, 1991; pages 47-56

Risk-factor Epidemiology: Science or Non-science?

Important associations, such as liver cirrhosis or Korsakoff's psychosis in alcoholism, retinopathy or foot gangrene in diabetes, aortic lesions or sabre tibias in syphilis, lung cancer in uranium ore miners, bladder cancer in workers with aniline dyes, are not discovered by epidemiologists but by clinicians, and they are not called 'associations' but the manifestations, signs, or complications of diseases which are their causes.

'Discoveries' of epidemiologists are of a more general nature. For example, to quote from the announcement of a conference on the prevention of cancer, which was organised by the Cancer Education Co-ordinating Group of the United Kingdom and Republic of Ireland, in association with the Health Education Authority, and held at the Royal Society of Medicine in London on November 21, 1989,

> A report commissioned by the European Commission found that one-third of all cancer deaths are attributable to cigarette smoking, one third could be attributable to diet including the consumption of alcohol, and another third are because of other factors including sexual and reproductive behaviour and occupational activities. The Committee of European Cancer Experts who produced the report recommend a 10 Point Code to help avoid the risk of developing cancers. The adoption of this Code by the public is the main aim of the "Europe Against Cancer" initiative.

Though there is some verbal hedging ('attributable' instead of 'caused'; 'could be' instead of 'is'), the message comes across loud and clear that the causes of cancer are well known and it is now up to the public to stop whingeing and start behaving. The message can be simplified, so that it is more easily remembered, as: 'smoking, drinking and sex are three main causes of cancer'. Other reputable epidemiologists are on record as saying that up to 70 per cent of all cancers are caused by diet. There is a certain plausibility in such claims, as it has been shown that there is a strong association between eating any of the three major constituents of the human diet (protein, fat, carbohydrate) and subsequent deaths, many of them from cancer.

The association game has three possible outcomes: positive association, negative association, or no association. As any of these three outcomes are generally deemed to be 'interesting', 'controversial', or 'in need of further research', they all get published. 'No association' is an uncommon outcome, since in most studies at least 'a tendency towards' a positive or negative association can be shown. Considering how many cancers exist, and how many items of diet can be entered into the game, the number of possible combinations is staggering and opens new vistas for the generations of epidemiologists to come. The scope of epidemiological research has been widened enormously by including 'passive' exposures to invisible electromagnetic waves, whether from home appliances, overhead wires, nuclear power stations or space, passive exposures to other people's smoke or to air pollutants (we inhale 20,000 litres of air a day!).

Associations nothing new, often random and seldom simple

As an example I shall use cabbage consumption, believed to be negatively associated with cancer, and coffee consumption, believed to be positively associated with heart disease. It is always tacitly understood, though rarely explicitly stated that 'association' implies in some way causation, since without such an understanding there would be no point in reporting a chance association. I am using cabbage as an example simply because I have just received the latest issue of Progress Against Cancer published by the Canadian Cancer Society, and on the last page there was the reproduction of a poster, issued by the Canadian Cancer Society, with the following text:

> Cancer Prevention. You can have a hand in it. The Canadian Cancer Society recommends that you include more vegetables from the cabbage family in your diet. These include brussel sprouts, broccoli and cauliflower. These vegetables may protect you against the risk of cancer.

This educational message is based on epidemiological research, but Cato the Elder (234-149 BC) wrote in his treatise *On Agriculture* that 'cabbage surpasses all other vegetables ... an ulcer of the breast and a cancer can be healed by the application of macerated cabbage'. Similarly, Dioscorides in *De materia medica* recommended direct application of cabbage on tumours to cause them to shrink. Apparently there is something in cabbage which has been exciting human minds for the past 2000 years.

There are snags, however. B N Ames and L S Gold found that cabbage is as strong a promoter of carcinogenesis as dioxin and that 'a 100-gram helping of broccoli might present roughly 20 times the possible hazard of the dioxin reference dose'.[3] To complicate matters even more, Marshall et al reported in their study of risk factors for cervical cancer that

> most notably, cruciferous vegetables [cabbage, coleslaw, turnips, but *not* broccoli] were associated with an *increased* [their emphasis] cervical cancer risk. The significance of the noted risk enhancement is greater than that of the protective effect of vitamin A. An earlier study indicated that cruciferous vegetable ingestion is protective against colon cancer. As noted then, there is abundant biochemical evidence that cruciferae could be protective in the gut, so that induction of aryl hydroxylase activity could be protective in the gut and carcinogenic in the lung and cervix.[4]

While there is no good reason to believe that cabbage has anything to do with cancer, it is characteristic of epidemiological literature that such chance associations as between cabbage in diet and mortality from some cancer are discussed in terms 'protective' or 'carcinogenic.'

Coffee drinking was always suspect as a 'risk factor.' King Charles issued a proclamation for the suppression of coffee houses in 1675, in which he

> commanded all manner of persons, that they or any of them do not presume from and after the tenth day of January next ensuing, to keep any public coffee house, or to utter or sell by retail, in his, her or their house or houses (to be spent

or consumed within the same) any coffee, chocolet, sherbett or tea, as they will answer the contrary at their utmost peril.

In 1695, the Medical School of Paris announced that coffee deprived men of their generative powers. Coffee drinkers, just like the victims of self-abuse, became shrivelled shadows of their former selves, with haggard looks and an uncontrollable tremor.

More recently, in 1988, a group of epidemiologists from the National Institute of Environmental Health Sciences at Research Triangle Park, North Carolina, reported in *The Lancet* that 'women who consumed more than the equivalent of one cup of coffee per day were half as likely to become pregnant as women who drank less'.[5] On the other hand, according to a news item in the *Daily Telegraph* of January 19, 1990, a study carried out among 744 people in Michigan, showed that those who drank coffee were full of beans, that is, they were more sexually active than those who did not drink coffee.

A group of epidemiologists from the Department of Health Services in Berkeley studied an association between coffee drinking and spontaneous abortions: results were inconclusive but suggestive of an association, particularly in women who suffered from the nausea of pregnancy. The authors concluded that 'further study is warranted'.

Scores of epidemiological studies have been devoted to analysing associations between coffee and bladder cancer, colorectal cancer, ovarian cancer, pancreatic cancer, kidney cancer, breast cancer, hypertension, hip fracture, pre-menstrual syndrome, and childhood diabetes. The list is not exhaustive. Bruce Ames reported that 'of 247 volatile natural chemicals reported in coffee (mostly pyrolysis products) 10 have been tested in chronic animal cancer tests and 7 are carcinogenic (eg furfural, catechol). The total amount of rodent carcinogens are roughly 9 mg/cup.'[8] However, the majority of studies on coffee and health have dealt with the risk of coronary heart disease in coffee drinkers. In a recent editorial in the *British Medical Journal* the editorialist reviewed 24 such studies.[9]

The plot has thickened since the most recent studies have exculpated caffeine and incriminated decaffeinated coffee instead. One of the chemicals used in the process of decaffeinisation is methylene chloride. This was shown to have a carcinogenic effect in rats who were administered methylene chloride at a dose of 1,000 mg/kg/day (equivalent of 24 million cups of decaffeinated coffee per day).[10] This does not quite explain the effect of coffee on heart disease, but, as the editorialist concluded 'before we can decide whether decaffeinated coffee increases the risk of heart disease longer studies with multiple assessment of exposure to decaffeinated and caffeinated coffee are needed'.

The new epidemiology provides justification for infinite research — and funding

The advantage of this approach is that one never gets a clear answer, which allows for studying the problem indefinitely. Alvin Weinberg, in discussing the probability of extremely improbable events (such as our examples of coffee causing various diseases, or cabbage causing or preventing cancer) introduced the concept of trans-science, by which he means problems which hang on the answers to questions which can be asked of science and yet which cannot be answered by science.[11]

In one of his examples, which is relevant for current epidemiological investigations into the effects of low-level radiation on health, the trans-scientific question was whether a 150 millirem dose of X-radiation would increase the spontaneous mutation rate in mice by 0.5 percent, as calculated by linear extrapolation from higher doses. To answer this question by a direct experiment would require 8 billion mice. And even if such an experiment could have been carried out, the relevance for humans would be unclear and the experiment would have to be repeated on eight billion men, to be sure!

As so many scares have been disseminated by epidemiological research into risk factors, further research is often called for to confirm or to deny the rumours. Recently, a group of American epidemiologists provided reassurance to vasectomised men that they are not at an increased risk of dying from heart disease. This will hold until other researchers will confirm the initial positive association.

When too many such conflicting observations have accumulated, a call is made for meta-analysis and possibly a consensus conference. As meta-analysis is increasingly used at consensus conferences, and invited meta-analysts conjure metaphysical 'statistical significance' from the insignificant, like the alchemists of old converting dross into false gold, the time will soon come for the metaconsensus of consensus.[12] In fact, earlier this year, the King Edward's Hospital Fund convened a meeting on consensus, and at one point they 'all agreed'.[13]

Risk factors largely irrelevant to search for causal mechanisms

The last official count of the risk factors for coronary heart disease was 246.[14] Since then many others have been discovered by assiduous epidemiologists. Some of them are listed in and compared with a selected list of risk factors for scurvy compiled before the cause of scurvy was known, that is the lack of vitamin C.[15]

Table 1: Risk factors for coronary heart disease and scurvy

Risk factors for coronary heart disease

age	divorced parents
male sex	illegitimate birth
mother tongue English	no church attendance
urban residence	Jewish religion
altitude	not being a Mormon
cold weather	alcoholism
noise	total abstinence
extramarital sex	obesity
snoring	slow beard growth
baldness	homocystinaemia
short stature	high blood sugar
not eating mackerel	low plasma zinc
no varsity athletics	no garlic
type A personality	high white cell count
work > 60 hrs/week	vasectomy

good financial status
low socioeconomic status
1-child family
being > 4th child
low education
intelligent wife
unlovingwife
non-supportive boss

early menopause
contraceptive pill
coffee
passive smoking
too much milk
too little milk
chlorinated water
widowhood

Risk factors for scurvy

bad butter
bad diet
copper boilers
debauchery
dejection
distilled spirits
fruit lack
gluttony
infection
mercury
spoiled flour
sugar

tobacco
unleavened bread
cold
dampness
external causes
inactivity
low marsh ground
sea air
season change
constitution
heredity
melancholy disposition

The plethora of risk factors leads some epidemiologists to postulate the so-called multifactorial aetiology. While in a certain sense, all events are multifactorial, even such trivial occurrences as being hit on the head with a chunk of frozen urine discarded from an overflying aircraft (the factors include: the speed of the aircraft, the speed and the direction of the wind, the time spent at a crossword during breakfast, the reason and the speed of the fatal walk, and myriads of others), we do not use the term 'multifactorial' when the cause of an event is understood.

Risk factors have nothing to do with causes. They are risk *markers*, but they are neither sufficient nor necessary to explain the risk. Thus, for example, the possession of a driving licence is a risk marker for death in a car accident, marshes are a risk marker for malaria, and homosexuality a risk marker for AIDS. The knowledge of risk factors rarely, if ever, contributes to the elucidation of causal mechanisms. At best, it may provide a hint as to where to look for the cause. When the cause of tuberculosis was still unknown, numerous risk factors were described, none of which was of any use to Koch in his laboratory studies leading to the discovery of the necessary cause — the mycobacterium.

It is the intimation by epidemiologists that they hold the key to the causes of diseases and their prevention which makes them overstep their brief and join the moralists in their preaching how to avoid death by being good, clean-living citizens.

The hope that by searching for risk factors, the causal mechanisms will somehow come to light is misplaced. Such an approach is the rich source of false leads. Thus, when the first cases of AIDS appeared in the USA, risk-factor epidemiologists looked at ethnic and religious background, alcohol and tobacco use, diet, residential and occupational histories, sexual practices and drug use. They concluded that the use of amyl nitrate ('poppers') was the strongest risk factor, implying a causal link.[16] The strength of association was of the same order as for smoking and lung cancer, yet this lead was a red herring.

Or, to use another example, when oestrogen-replacement therapy was thought to be a risk factor for coronary heart disease, two 'definitive' studies were published in the same issue of the prestigious *New England Journal of Medicine*: one showed a significant negative association, and the other, a significant positive association, implying causative or protective mechanisms. It would be reasonable to conclude that at least one of these epidemiological studies was wrong, and possibly both. The accompanying editorial was painful reading.[17] The editorialist admitted that both studies 'appeared to be methodologically sound'. The most likely explanation for the disagreement between the two studies was that such studies and by implication the results of countless other observational studies, are subject to a great deal more variability than is captured by the usual kinds of statistical tests and confidence limits. I simply cannot tell from present evidence whether these hormones add to the risk of various cardiovascular diseases, diminish the risk, or leave it unchanged, and must resort to the investigator's great cop-out: more research is needed.[18]

This kind of 'science' is not exactly Nobel prize stuff.

In conclusion

Alvan Feinstein, casting a cool eye at some of the nonsense going on in the name of risk-factor epidemiology, suggested that until the new paradigms, methods, and data are developed, non-epidemiological scientists and members of the lay public will have to use common sense and their own scientific concepts to evaluate the reported evidence.[19]

Notes and References

1 Lilienfeld DE. Definitions of epidemiology.
   American Journal of Epidemiology 1978; 107: 87-90.

2. Canadian Cancer Society, *Progress Against Cancer*, Vol.44, No. 1, 1991.

3. Ames BN and Gold LS. Misconceptions regarding environmental pollution and cancer causation. In: Moore M ed. Health Risks and the Media: Perspectives on Media Coverage of Risk Assessment and Health. American Medical Association, Chicago, 1989: 19-34.

4. Marshall JR, Graham S, Byers T, Swanson M, Brasure J. Diet and smoking in the epidemiology of cancer of the cervix.
   Journal of the National Cancer Institute 1983; 70: 847-851.

5. *The Lancet*, 24 December, 1988, 1453.

6. *The Daily Telegraph*, 19 January, 1990.

7. *American Journal of Epidemiology* 1990; 132: 796.

8. Ames BN. Endogenous vs. exogenous factors as major cancer risk determinants. *Proceedings of the American Association for Cancer Research* 1990 ;31: 512-513.

9. *British Medical Journal*, 6 April, 1991, 804.

10. Morris DH. Decaffeination of coffee. *Journal of the American Medical Association* 1985; 254: 825.

11. Weinberg AM. Science and trans-science. *Minerva* 1972; 10: 207-222.

12. Skrabanek P. Nonsensus consensus. *The Lancet* 1990; 335: 1446-1447.

13. *British Medical Journal*, 6 April 1991, 800.

14. Hopkins PN and Williams RP. A survey of 246 suggested coronary risk factors. *Atherosclerosis* 1981; 40: 1-52.

15. Klevay LM. The role of copper, zinc and other chemical elements in ischemic heart disease. In: Rennert OM and Chan WY eds. Metabolism of Metals in Man. CRC Press, New York,1984: 129.

16. Vandenbroucke JP, Pardoel VPAM. An autopsy of epidemiological methods: the case of "poppers" in the early epidemic of the acquired immunodeficiency syndrome (AIDS). *American Journal of Epidemiology* 1989; 129: 455-457.

17. Bailar JC. When research results are in conflict. *New England Journal of Medicine* 1985; 313: 1080-1081.

18. Feinstein AR. Scientific standards in epidemiological studies of the menace of daily life. *Science* 1988; 242: 1257-1263

12

SMOKING AND SOCIETY

1. The ideology of anti-smoking campaigns

> To be a libertine is a physical condition like
> that of a morphinist, a drunkard or a smoker.
>
> L.N. Tolstoy, *The Kreutzer Sonata*

Smoking, together with drinking and fornication, has always been a mote in the eye of the virtuous. Throughout the ages, the preachers in their commendable attempts to root out vice from society threatened the errant souls with the fire of hell, and when possible, buttressed their claim that the wages of sin is death with medical evidence. But many sinners were beyond redemption: Jean Cocteau observed that to preach to an addict that he would feel much better if he kicked his enslaving habit was like telling Tristan to kill Isolde, which would make him feel much better afterwards. Another obstacle in winning the battle against evil was that the Devil was painted blacker than he was, and many instinctively disbelieved it.

Pleasurable vices, such as smoking, are, undoubtedly, at times rewarded by disease and death. But a cynic may observe that life itself is an incurable, sexually transmitted disease, even for the virtuous. The knowledge that cigarettes are bad for health is not recent: Eric Partridge in his Dictionary of Slang dates the colloquial term 'coffin nails' for cigarettes as early as 1885. This was not a term coined by a Surgeon General but by ordinary folk. The First World War slang for cigarettes was 'gaspers'. Yet it was also part of common experience that the majority of smokers escaped the more gruesome penalties. The popular image of a pipe smoker was, and still is, an old man, and not someone cut down in his prime. Most smokers do not die from lung cancer, and the majority of the minority so afflicted leave this world in

---

First published in 'Other People's Tobacco Smoke'. A K Armitage (Ed). Galen Press, 1991.

their old age. Even if all cancer of the lung disappeared by magic, average life expectancy would be extended by 6 months at most. For those who fear death, any extension of life means the corresponding extension of the duration of their fear. There are other diseases to which smokers are prone, such as coronary heart disease, but this does not have the same potential for instilling dread into a smoker as cancer has; it is correspondingly less used in anti-smoking propaganda; as a cynic may answer, give me that any time rather than Alzheimer's dementia.

In Western democracies, lip service is still being paid to Mill's concept of liberty, which embodies the principle that no one is warranted in saying to another that he shall not do with his life what he chooses, and intense intellectual activity is directed to producing sound counter-arguments against this preposterous thesis. Traditionally, there has been a certain reluctance to outlaw private behaviour considered to have no function other than that of providing pleasure, mainly because of the lesson taught by the fiasco of Prohibition. Widespread vices such as drinking, fornication and smoking are as difficult to abolish by decree as the law of gravity. Thus the present policy of tobacco-phobes has been a pragmatic compromise between the aspiration towards total prohibition and its practicality. For a start, smokers may be discriminated against when applying for a job, seeking insurance, or when in need of medical treatment. Their habit is alternately described as a disease and an irresponsibility. But it is not easy to prevent people from lighting up, provided they do it in designated areas, unless it can also be shown that they harm not only themselves but also other people near them. This is the innocent-bystander argument, used with great effect in debates leading to Prohibition.

2. The history of the war against tobacco

> Tobacco has nowhere been forbidden in the Bible, but then it had not yet been discovered ... It was possible that God knew Paul would have forbidden smoking, and had purposely arranged the discovery of tobacco for a period at which Paul

should no longer be living.

Samuel Butler: *The Way of all Flesh*

The present war against smoking is not just 25 years old, as the US Surgeon General would have us believe. The earlier battles against tobacco are worth recalling in order to see the present blitzkrieg within a historical context, rather than as the result of some new 'scientific' discovery of tobacco as an evil.

Within a year of his accession to the English throne, King James I wrote a short, rambling tract against smoking, entitled A *Counterblaste to Tobacco* (1604). The last sentence of this curious pamphlet is still a favourite quote of modern anti-tobacco crusaders:

> 'A custome lothsome to the eye, hatefull to the nose, harmefull to the braine, daungerous to the lungs, and in the blacke stinking fume thereof, neerest resembling the horrible Stigian smoke of the pit that is bottomlesse.'

It says it all, neatly combining the Government health warning with moral damnation, and is probably the first reference to the noxiousness of ETS.

Perusal of the *Counterblaste* makes it clear that the King's concern was not for the welfare of his subjects, but rather for his own welfare. James argued that idle delights and soft delicacies, among which he ranked smoking, were 'the first seeds of subversion of all great monarchies', and showed apprehension lest his subjects become disabled by smoking and thus be prevented from discharging their duty to defend with their bodies 'the maintenance both of the honour and safetie of their King and Commonwealth.' The King feared that 'there cannot be a more base, and yet hurtfull, corruption in a Countrey, than is the vile use (or abuse) of taking Tobacco in this Kingdome.'

In 1605, anxious to have his assault against tobacco endorsed by Academia, James invited himself to a public debate at Oxford University on the harm of smoking. Not surprisingly, dons concurred with the King that the use of tobacco should be excluded from the habits of all sensible men and banned in medical schools. There was only one physician who dared to contradict the King's wisdom: a Dr Cheynell, who had graduated from the medical school only two years previously, took the floor and, puffing on his pipe, opposed the King. Fortunately for him, he expressed himself so wittily that the King laughed, and Cheynell, as a court jester, survived. The King then went to Cambridge, where appropriate precautions were taken by the Vice-Chancellor who ordered that neither staff nor students should smoke or take snuff during the King's visit. But even James I realised that the imposition of heavy import duties on tobacco would be more beneficial to him than issuing a prohibition order; Cardinal Richelieu gave the same advice in 1629 to the French monarch, who hated smokers.

The attitude of the Church to smoking moved quickly from abhorrence to toleration. In 1642, Pope Urban VIII issued an anti-tobacco bull, *Ad futuram rei memoriam*, in which he denounced the use of tobacco by the clergy:

'We blush to state that during the actual celebration of Holy Mass, the priests do not shrink from taking tobacco through the mouth or nostrils, thus soiling the altar linen and infecting the churches with its noxious fumes.'

He threatened with instant excommunication anyone using tobacco in church. His successor, Pope Innocent X, upheld the ban, but the next pope, Benedict X, quashed Innocent's ban and ordered it to be 'withdrawn, annulled, and utterly repealed, as though it had never existed.' Benedict had become enamoured with nicotine himself and the Papacy allowed the sale of tobacco and brandy, provided that the contractors paid a reasonable revenue to the Papal states.

In less enlightened parts of the world, smokers were persecuted for their monstrous crime. For example, in 1633, the Ottoman sultan, Murad IV, made smoking a capital offence. Reports (not well authenticated) indicate that his father, Ahmed, used to punish the wretches caught smoking in public by having a pipe-stem thrust through their nose and, as a warning to discourage others, had them paraded through the streets on a donkey. Murad IV, reasoning along the same lines as James I, thought that smoking sapped the fighting ability of his soldiers, and he further thought that smoking made men infertile, (this side-effect was rediscovered by antismoking campaigners quite recently), thus reducing the future military potential of the Ottoman armies. Soldiers caught smoking on the battlefield were dealt with summarily by beheading, quartering, or just having their hands and feet crushed and being left to their fate. Even such savagery was not enough to stem the inexorable spread of the tobacco habit and Murad IV's successor became a passionate smoker.

In 17th century Russia, the tsars had a policy of punishing smokers by slitting their lips or nostrils, or, in the case of tobacco sellers, flogging them to death or castration. In Denmark, in 1655, the Court Physician, Simon Paulli, wrote a denunciation of smoking at the request of Christian IV, King of Denmark and Norway. In Japan, in 1616, the property of smokers was liable to confiscation, and a Chinese law of 1638 threatened tobacco sellers with decapitation.

In England, however, smoking very quickly became widespread and respectable; it was even believed that smoking protected against the plague. In 1665, at Eton, all the boys were obliged to smoke every morning, and Tom Rogers, who was a yeoman beadle at Eton, recalled that he was never whipped so much in his life as he was one morning for not smoking. The editor of *The Medical Press*, writing in 1899, when boys were flogged for smoking, observed that a boy is a curious animal:

> 'This goes to prove that when doctors deal with boys, they should prescribe in exact opposition to their wishes in order to give a fair chance to the science of medicine.'

Health educators of youth, please take note!

Elsewhere, tobacco was available only on a doctor's prescription, as in Germany and Bavaria after the Thirty Years War. This idea was revived in 1983 by Dr Kilcoyne of the Irish Heart Foundation who called for a register of all smokers in Ireland, so that no-one could smoke unless registered; and in 1976, Mr George Teeling-Smith, director of the UK Office of Health Economics, suggested that cigarettes should be available only on prescription.

In 1667, the burgomaster of Zurich ordered that smokers be put to forced labour or banished. A German preacher, Jacob Balde, wrote in 1658: 'What difference is there between a smoker and a suicide, except that one takes longer to kill himself than the other.' In 1699, the President of the Paris School of Medicine declared that the act of love was a brief epileptic fit, while smoking was a permanent epilepsy. (A few years ago in an editorial in the *Journal of the American Medical Association*, Feb. 28, 1986, smoking was described as 'making love with death').

The revival of anti-smoking propaganda in the 19th century had the character of a crusade in which doctors and moralists joined hands. Expanding capitalist industry required masses of workers whose efficiency was not impaired by tobacco or alcohol. In Victorian England, human weaknesses were seen as a threat to the accumulation of capital, especially when indulged in by the working class. The puritanical spirit of the Victorians may be glimpsed in regulations issued to office workers in Lichfield in 1852, which, among other prohibitions, specified that 'the craving for tobacco, wines and spirits is a human weakness, and, as such, is forbidden to all members of the clerical staff.' This was in the era when small children were exploited in coal mines, often spending 12-14 hours a day underground, without objection from the medical and church authorities who backed the newly-formed anti-tobacco leagues and societies.

Rarely, a tone of moderation was sounded in the medical press. In 1833, James Johnson, the editor of the *Medico-Chirurgical Review*, expressed doubts about the alarmist reports from Germany that tobacco was responsible for 50% of all deaths among men between the ages of 18 and 25. Johnson wrote that while smoking may be a beastly and intolerable custom, it is 'not as pernicious as those who dislike it would seem to imagine', and he tried to dispel the fears that London's air was strongly poisoned by tobacco smoke, by pointing out that it would 'require many more pipes than are at present in circulation to sully the smoky air of the modern Babylon.'

The 1850s in Britain were dominated by The Great Tobacco Debate.

This was triggered by an article in the *Lancet* in 1856 by Samuel Solly, FRS, Surgeon to St. Thomas's Hospital in London, who argued that the recently observed increase in cases of paralysis was caused by smoking. Correspondent after correspondent enumerated all the kinds of diseases caused by smoking, including muscular debility, jaundice, cancers of the tongue, lip and throat, the tottering knee, trembling hands, softening of the brain, epilepsy, impairment of the intellect, insanity, impotence, spermatorrhoea, apoplexy, mania, cretinism, diseases of the pancreas and liver, deafness, bronchitis, and heart disease. Others added that tobacco harmed not only the smoker but also his offspring. A Dr Pidduck wrote in the *Lancet* on February 14, 1856:

> 'The enervation, the hypochondriasis, the hysteria, the insanity, the dwarfish deformities, the suffering lives and early deaths of the children of inveterate smokers bear ample testimony to the feebleness and unsoundness of the constitution transmitted by this pernicious habit.'

Worries were expressed that the health of England was at stake and that smoking would reduce the English race in the scale of nations to a point which approached the national degeneracy of the Turks. One correspondent pointed out that the constant use of tobacco in Germany made spectacles as much part and parcel of a German as a hat was of an Englishman, and concluded that a careful comparison of morbidity and mortality among smokers and non-smokers would clearly show that nicotine, tar and scores of other poisons in tobacco, shorten life.

Common sense, as usual, was in short supply, but one correspondent warned that exaggeration was counterproductive: a psychiatrist, J.C. Bucknill, observed that:

> 'The arguments applied against moderate use of tobacco are of the same one-sided, inconclusive kind as those which teetotallers have adduced against the enjoyment of fermented drinks. They employ the same fallacy — that because a thing is not necessary for the maintenance of

> health, and because its abuse is sometimes the cause of disease, therefore its use is pernicious and objectionable under all circumstances.'

The editor of the *Lancet* at one point in The Great Debate also warned against overstating the case, with the unwanted consequence of losing 'our permanent hold upon the mind of the public, as the moral razzia does not know where to stop and raves now against tobacco, now against meat, salt, alcohol, or sugar.' The editorial posed the question, 'Are poetry, painting, port wine, and pipes to be run down by a moral razzia, and humanity with all its innumerable cravings and capacities for enjoyment, reduced to the condition of an intellectual vegetable?' The public generally shared this sentiment and remained largely unimpressed by the anti-smoking tirades. A barrister, A. Steinmetz, wrote a pamphlet defending the smokers and accused Solly of suffering from the ex-smoker's syndrome. Steinmetz also asked: 'Do they really expect to persuade the public to believe that they, the doctors, feel interested in the continued health of nations?' The same question can legitimately be asked today.

3. The 20th century : the final battle?

> 'Science has demonstrated that (tobacco) is a poison; that (tobacco) is a habit-forming drug that shackles millions of our citizens and maintains slavery in our midst; that it lowers in a fearful way the standard of efficiency of the Nation, reducing enormously the national wealth, entailing startling burdens of taxation; .... attacks the young when they are entitled to protection; undermines public health, slaughtering, killing and wounding our citizens many times more than war, pestilence and famine combined; that blights the progeny of the Nation...'

I have deceived the reader slightly by substituting in this quote the word 'tobacco' for 'alcohol'. The text comes from a speech by Richmond Hobson from Alabama introducing the Prohibition resolution in the US House of Representatives on December 22, 1914. Let us compare this excerpt with the modern 'scientific' view of smoking, as presented in an editorial in the *Journal of the American Medical Association* of April 11, 1986:

> 'Smoking is exacting a heavier toll in lives and dollars than cocaine, heroin, AIDS, traffic accidents, murder, and terrorist attacks combined; the citizens of this country are losing their lives to tobaccoism at the rate of 1000 per day. At this rate we will lose 6 million of our brothers and sisters during the next 16 years and 4 months, that is by the year of 2000.'

The preacher's condescension in his use of 'brothers and sisters' is noteworthy. The comparison in the editorial to the 6 million victims of the Holocaust is in bad taste, to put it mildly.

The intoxication with numbers is another characteristic of the modern crusaders against smoking. They typically use big population blocks as denominators to obtain bigger and bigger numbers. Richard Peto, a leading anti-smoking exponent and a statistician, announced that 'of all children alive today in China under the age of 20 years, 50 million will eventually be killed by tobacco.' This would put the hecatombs of the Second World War in the shade. The *British Medical Journal*, referring to another such statistic, 'typical of the Oxford epidemiologist Richard Peto', quoted that 'about 20 million children now living in Europe will be killed by tobacco in their middle age.' And *The Times* reported on January 1, 1988, that according to Mrs Edwina Currie, 'more than a million schoolchildren and 60,000 babies born this year will die of smoking-related diseases such as lung cancer.' Surprisingly, no-one has yet used the population of the whole world as a denominator: this would produce numbers of babies, toddlers, schoolchildren, and other children, killed by tobacco in truly phenomenal ranges. Perhaps the reason for this reticence is the fear of overkill.

Dr J.H. Jaffe, a psychiatrist whom Richard Nixon put in charge of the war on 'drugs' in 1969, declared smoking a mental disorder—a modern euphemism for the 'degeneracy' of 19th century smokers. In the total war against smoking now waged, any ruse, stratagem, or tactic is allowed and encouraged. According to a booklet published by the

British Medical Association in 1986 and entitled appropriately 'Smoking Out the Barons', anti-smoking campaigners should use any means at their disposal to scare or scandalise the public and the smokers. One of the instructions reads: 'If you have time when nothing much happens (or everything goes wrong), bring some eminent figure, clever stunt, or scandalous data.'

The list of diseases and woes ready to descend on those who smoke is even longer than the list of the Great Debate of 1856, with hardly any overlap. It now includes conditions and diseases such as hip fractures, stroke, subalveolar breast abcess, leukaemia, infertility, menstrual disorders, varicocele, migraine, peptic ulcer, hearing loss, pulmonary embolism, Alzheimer's dementia, hypertension, and all kinds of cancer, including the cancer of the penis and cervix, breast, liver and kidney. Children of smokers are said to be of low intelligence and slower in school, and prone to asthma, pneumonia, bronchitis, meningitis, ear infections, lung cancer, hyperactivity, leukaemia, various cancers, and cot death. Women who smoke in pregnancy are threatened with the possibility that their children, if not stillborn, will be born with a cleft palate or will have other congenital abnormalities, and their physical and mental health will be impaired. Women who live with smokers will get cervical cancer or breast cancer, though some will die of heart attack. The media bring new scares regularly, and for an ordinary reader it has become impossible to distinguish nonsense from a genuine warning. I have heard one woman saying that she read so much about smoking and disease that she decided to give up reading. Health educators despair that people still believe that cancer is an incurable disease. What else can they believe if cancer is used as a synonym for death to scare away smokers? As the bogey of cancer tends to evoke fatalistic inertia in the listeners, the anti-smoking propagandists have been experimenting with exploitation of concern about self-image, hoping that it might be more effective. For example, the statement that smokers are impotent 'could be a powerful encouragement in programmes to decrease prevalence in smoking', wrote two researchers in the *Lancet* on March 9, 1985. One of the oldest canards is that smoking 'cures' and wrinkles the skin. In Ben Johnson's

Bartholomew Fayre (1614), Justice Overdo warns that tobacco makes the smoker's complexion like the Indian's that vends it, besides 'turning his lung rotten, the liver spotted, and the brain smoked like the backside of the pigwoman's booth.' This is now known as 'fag-fiend's face' (according to a headline in *The Guardian*) and the pressure group ASH (Action for Smoking and Health) has been using this in its anti-smoking propaganda, hoping that it may reach women in particular, as 'smoker's face' is said to be commoner among them. In 1985, the British Medical Journal even published a gallery of mug shots of inveterate smokers to show how ugly they were. H.L. Mencken, in his *Americana* collection of newspaper clippings from the 1920s, assembled for the delectation of connoisseurs of the preposterous, included one which claimed that smoking makes women's noses red and causes moustaches to grow.

The last campaign which preceded the present one waged by the US Surgeon General and his troops was the fascist anti-smoking movement. As the correspondent of the *Journal of the American Medical Association* reported from Germany on August 3, 1939, a professor of public health addressed a mass rally attended by 15,000 people on the evils of alcohol and tobacco. He stated that tobacco was highly injurious to health and reduced the number of those fit for military service. (Note the echoes of James I and Murad IV.) He pointed out further that there was a close connection between cigarette smoking and physical and mental susceptibility to disease and to disturbances of the normal sexual life. He promised that tobacco addiction would be mercilessly combated by the government and that 'increasingly shameful methods of advertising' by the tobacco industry, in which smoking was linked with manliness, sport, and car-driving, would not be tolerated. Hermann Goering, the Commander-in-Chief of the Nazi Air Force, forbade his pilots to smoke in public, on marches, or in brief periods off duty. And Hitler himself, in 1942, gave 100,000 DM of his own personal funds as a contribution to the Institute for the Struggle Against Tobacco at the University of Jena. Hitler confided to his personal physician on March 11, 1942, that:

> I am convinced that if I had been a smoker I would never

have been able to bear the cares and anxieties which have been a burden to me for so long. Perhaps the German people owes its salvation to the fact. So many outstanding men have been lost to me through tobacco poisoning.'

In Iraq, a country accused of using chemical weapons against its own population and of torturing children, the first anti-smoking day was launched on October 28, 1987. All government and public agencies participated by Presidential decree, and a further decree prohibited smoking at all government and political party meetings and functions. This great contribution to public health in Iraq was applauded by the International Cancer News.

Even in Western democracies, the present anti-smoking campaigns are more an expression of single issue fanaticism which animates various pressure groups than a genuine concern about the health of individuals. In the United States, which stands as a world leader in combating the evil of tobacco, the child poverty rate increased from 16% in 1979 to 20% in 1987, as documented in *Science* by Professor T.M. Smedding from the Vanderbilt Institute for Public Policy, and B. B. Torrey from the US Bureau of Census.

The issue of environmental tobacco smoke (ETS) came to be of central importance to the anti-smoking activists, for if it could be shown that it was a health hazard, then smokers could be branded not only as social misfits, but also as murderers. In 1911, Dr Herbert Tidswell (an ex-smoker, like many of his kin) argued that:

> 'A pregnant woman should never be exposed to the risk of inhaling or absorbing tobacco smoke, lest it should injure the foetus. It is dangerous for a pregnant woman to be in a room where a person is smoking, or has been recently smoking ...The exposure to tobacco smoke may retard development of the foetus, induce various congenital diseases or even abortions.'

Despite these dire forebodings, anti-smoking campaigners have not succeeded so far in providing scientific evidence that ETS is a health hazard. This is not to dispute that ETS is a nuisance to some non-smokers, and occasionally also to smokers themselves. Even in the official anti-smoking literature, the weakness of the evidence is admitted, with some reluctance. The official estimates suggest that a non-smoker who lives with a smoker may increase his or her risk of lung cancer from 0.010% (if he were not exposed to any ETS) to 0.012% annually. That is, instead of 10 nonsmokers dying of lung cancer out of 100,000 non-smokers not exposed to ETS, living with the smoker increases this risk by 20% (the actual estimates give a range of 10% to 30%) to 12 deaths from lung cancer among 100,000 non-smokers. Some epidemiologists find this glass-bead game exciting, but for experienced observers this looks more like an idle pastime. For example, the editor of the *International Journal of Epidemiology*, Dr Charles Du Ve Florey, wrote recently in his journal that 'the passive smoking literature is littered with inconclusive studies ... there seems to be occasional significant observations which hint at a real effect, but until more data are to hand, the interpretation may reflect more the authors' point of view or degree of scientific caution' —in other words, their wishful thinking. This extreme degree of uncertainty is hardly ever conveyed by the media to the reader, who is led to believe that innocent bystanders are being killed in large numbers. In some of the studies it has even been shown that passive smoking is more harmful than active smoking!

I cannot here review all the studies on ETS and health, but one example may suffice as an illustration. In the February 1989 issue of the *American Journal of Public Health*, researchers from the National Institute of Environmental Health Sciences and from Johns Hopkins University recorded deaths from all causes in non-smokers who lived with smokers. The risk of exposure to ETS was the same as the risk of active smoking of less than 10 cigarettes a day, both risks being indistinguishable from the risk to non-smokers not exposed to ETS. As a non-smoker exposed to ETS inhales about 1% of the smoke which the active smoker inhales, this would mean that to smoke 10 cigarettes equals exposure to the smoke from 1000 cigarettes, neither of which had a demonstrable effect on mortality. What was even more interesting in this study was the observation that the frequency of cancer deaths was exactly the same in non-smokers, whether or not they were exposed to ETS. Common sense suggests that, even if there were a risk from exposure to ETS, it would be so small as to be undetectable.

The war against tobacco is not the last. Clarence Seward Darrow, the famous US lawyer and defender of civil liberties, argued in 1909 that the prohibitionists could not care less about the welfare of the poor and used their fundamentalist rhetoric for diverting attention from poverty and injustice. He characterised their tactics when challenged about their real concern for the health of others: "Let's first destroy Rum. Join with us on a moral issue. Let us get rid of Rum and then we will help you'. And if you help them get rid of rum and go back you will find these gentlemen in a corner and they will say: 'Not now. Let us get rid of tobacco. Let us get rid of theatres and cards and billiards and dancing and everything else, and then we will attend to you."

In conclusion, to preclude any misrepresentation of this chapter as the covert defence of a detestable habit, let me close with the words of the ageing Luis Bunuel, from his autobiography *Mon Dernier Soupir*.

> 'My dear reader, let me conclude my reflexions on alcohol and tobacco, those promoters of lasting friendships and fertile inspiration, with this twofold counsel: do not drink and do not smoke; it is bad for your health.'

Further reading

Count Corti. *A History of smoking*. London: Harrap, London, 1931.

Compton Mackenzie. *Sublime Tobacco*. Chatto & Windus, London, 1957.

Walker RB. Medical aspects of tobacco smoking and the anti-tobacco movement in Britain in the nineteenth century. *Medical History* 1980; 24: 391-402.

Tollison RD. *Smoking and Society. Towards a more balanced assessment.* Lexington Books, DC Heath & Co, Massachusetts, 1986.

13

THE POVERTY OF EPIDEMIOLOGY

A perusal of the abstracts of papers presented at the twenty-third annual meeting of the Society for Epidemiological Research at Snowbird, Utah (June 12-15, 1990) [1], made me wonder whether epidemiology, in the absence of epidemics, is not a misnomer for scaremongering made respectable by the use of sophisticated statistical methods, and whether one of the reasons for this state of affairs is not a high prevalence of epidemiologists when the incidence of problems soluble by epidemiological methods is low.

It would seem that any combination of "exposure" and disease, regardless of biological implausibility, or even without any underlying hypothesis, is fair game for calculating relative risks, odds ratios, or proportional hazards. The association game has three possible outcomes: positive association, negative association, or no association. As any of these three outcomes is generally thought to be "interesting," "controversial," or just "in need of further research," they all get published. Combining these three possible outcomes with any two combinations of a potential risk factor (traditionally, sexual behaviour, alcohol drinking, and smoking, but now including any pleasurable activity, be it idleness, eating, or coffee drinking), the game has more possible combinations than Cluedo. The scope of epidemiological research has been enormously widened by including "passive" exposures to invisible electromagnetic waves, whether from home appliances, overhead wires, X-ray machines, or space, "passive" exposures to other people's smoke or other air pollutants, "passive" exposures to innumerable food additives, and other menaces of everyday life.

This paper first appeared in *Perspectives in Biology and Medicine*, 35, 2, Winter 1992. © 1992 by the University of Chicago. All rights reserved.
Reproduced by kind permission of the University of Chicago Press.

The Poverty of Epidemiology

Three groups of researchers looked at male breast cancer, a relatively uncommon disorder. According to one abstract, more than three medical X-rays increased the risk. Another study lent "support to the theory that exposure to electromagnetic fields may be related to [male] breast cancer". This was contradicted by a third study, in which no effect of occupational exposure to electromagnetic fields on breast cancer in males was observed, but the study was not altogether negative: widowed and never-married men had an increased risk, as shown by "unconditional logistic regression modelling." We are not one iota wiser, although the general feeling lingers that some radiation in some organisms may increase the risk of some cancers. As pointed out by Weinberg [2], trans-scientific questions are those that can be asked of science but cannot be answered by science, such as whether the amount of electromagnetic energy to which we are normally exposed increases the risk of cancer. In one of his examples, a study of the spontaneous mutation rate in mice exposed to 150 millirem of X-rays would require 8 billion mice in order to show an increase of one half percent (as extrapolated from much higher radiation doses, assuming a linear regression). Or perhaps 8 billion men, as extrapolation from mice to men is tricky. In other words, a potentially answerable question is unanswerable in real life.

As so many scares have been disseminated by epidemiological research and avidly taken up by the media, who could hardly be blamed, further research is deemed necessary to confirm or deny previous reports. This time, one abstract provided reassurance to vasectomised men that they are not at an increased risk of dying of heart disease. This will hold until another report contradicts this. When too many such conflicting observations have accumulated a call is made for metaanalysis, that is, pooling studies with not quite the same methodologies and not quite the same populations, in hope that if none of them made much sense, the sum total will throw light on the matter.

Women have been harassed more than men by epidemiologists, on account of having two sexual organs of interest: the uterus and the breast. Contraceptive pills "may have a substantial impact on incidence of invasive cervical cancer" was a conclusion of one abstract (though the verb "may" implies that the opposite may also be true), particularly if they do not eat tomatoes, since, according to another abstract, "increased odds of [cervical intraepithelial neoplasia] were associated with decreased consumption of tomatoes (p = 0.02)". In another abstract, "dark yellow-orange vegetables" (carrots?) were recommended as a prophylactic agent against cancer of the vulva (orally, not topically!). Coffee drinking appeared in an unusual context (the main variations have been rehearsed before): could it cause spontaneous abortions? The answer was yes and no: the overall risk was not significant, but in a subgroup of women with nausea the risk was increased. Not surprisingly, the authors suggested that "further study is warranted to examine the interaction between nausea and caffeine," provided a sponsor can be found. The results could be interesting as there are three possible outcomes: no association—which would be controversial; negative association—which would be controversial; or positive association —which would confirm a controversial finding.

Electromagnetism is a rewarding field of research as it can be measured and it is ubiquitous. One study investigated the effect of "periconceptual use" of electric blankets or "heated waterbeds" (an American equivalent of the hot-water bottle?). This could have serious implications in Ireland, where bedrooms have been traditionally unheated and icy cold as a cheap substitute for unavailable contraception. Fortunately, no association was found between bed warmers and cleft palate with or without cleft lip, anencephalus, or spina bifida. It was also reassuring to find that electric blankets were not incriminated in breast cancer, despite the fact that the use of electric blankets "leads to relatively high exposure to electromagnetic fields to the area of the pineal gland," believed to be the seat of soul by Descartes. And yet another study looked at alcohol and breast cancer; this time it drew a blank.

"The effect of depression on stroke incidence has not been previously examined." This is hard to believe, but some combinations have been overlooked. "Cox proportional hazards regression analysis indicated that [depression] scores were predictive of stroke in the univariate analysis, but were not predictive of stroke in a model with control variables." Conclusion: "The implication of these results for future research are discussed." Depressing, isn't it?

And what about a report showing that "cardiovascular disease has overall protective effect" against traffic accidents among drivers? Would a national diet of three eggs a day reduce carnage on roads? Have you fastened your seat belt and buttered your toast?

Smoking is not good for health. The surgeon-general has more than 50,000 references to prove it. The Utah meeting enriched the literature further: Cigarette smoking was a risk factor for *hip fracture*. A causal association was found between smoking and *pelvic inflammatory disease*, which may lead to *ectopic pregnancy* and *tubal infertility*. Paternal smoking was associated with an increased risk of *ventricular septal defect, hydrocephalus, urethral stenosis, mouth cyst,* and *Bell's palsy*. Maternal smoking and *cleft lip* with or without *cleft palate* was difficult to evaluate as there was "a marked heterogeneity across recognised subclassification of cleft lip." However, an association between maternal smoking and strabismus was quite strong, especially among infants weighing more than 3,500 g. Smoking in pregnancy also increased the risk of *abruptio placentae*. More generally, smoking was found to be a risk factor for *fire injuries* in households, and for *cataract*. I was reminded of the Great Smoking Debate in the *Lancet* in 1856, which spanned many months in the correspondence columns.

The following associations, believed to be causal, of smoking and disease were among those reported by observant general practitioners, albeit without the benefit of modern statistical methods: the tottering knee, trembling hands, softening of the brain, infertility, epilepsy, jaundice, insanity, cretinism, stroke, spermatorrhoea, deafness, and impairment of intellect.

Following the critique by Feinstein [3] of the poverty of epidemiological methods ("despite peer-review approval, the current methods need substantial improvement to produce trustworthy scientific evidence"), we should also look at what is being studied by these methods. The subject matter does not inspire trust either.

References

1. *Am. J Epidemiol* 1990; 132: 752-826.

2. Weinberg AM. Science and transcience. *Minerva* 1972;10:207-222.

3. Feinstein A. Scientific standards in epidemiological studies of the menace of daily life. *Science* 1988; 242: 1257-1263.

14

THE EMPTINESS OF THE BLACK BOX

The "black box" strategy is a current paradigm of epidemiologic research, better described by the term "risk factor epidemiology". In the hope of unraveling causes of diseases, associations are sought between disease and various "exposures". "Black box" is an untested postulate linking the exposure and the disease in a causal sequence. An association, by itself a fortuitous finding, is thus converted, by logical sleight-of-hand, into a causal link. The causal mechanism remains unknown ("black"), but its existence is implied ("box"). Advocates of this strategy see it as a "unique virtue" of epidemiology[1] and the source of "the most important findings [of cancer causation] thus far .... The 'black box' strategy looks at the cancers that people chiefly die of and then looks for populations (defined by country or county of residence, by dietary, drinking or smoking habits, by religion, occupation, or reproduction, and by many other aspects of people's life-style or environment) which differ in their death rates from these cancers to determine what seem to be the chief manipulable determinants [= causes] of today's cancers."[2]

Its detractors believe that this strategy is an embarrassing liability.[3-6] As there are no underlying hypotheses for this kind of "research", beyond a general feeling that "diseases of civilisation" are caused by civilization, the method is based on "stabs in the dark" (in Savitz's terminology), by which various "biologically vague but important circumstances," such as life-style, are randomly linked to various chronic diseases. Items of diet, for example, are played against various cancers, in the hope of discovering causes. Senior risk factor epidemiologists are on record as stating that the main "causes" of cancer have already been discovered by the "black box" strategy, namely, smoking,

---

This paper first appeared in *Epidemiology*, 1994; 5: 553-555

© 1994 Epidemiology Resources Inc. Reproduced by kind permission of Lippincott, Williams and Wilkins

alcohol consumption, sexual behaviour, and bad diets.

The aim of science is to find universal laws governing the world around us and within us; it is about dismantling the "black box." It is doubtful whether anything is ever discovered by "stabs in the dark." In science, at least, one proceeds from an interesting problem, embedded within a larger body of systematized knowledge, toward its solution or rejection. Reasoning, such as "the existence of cars is associated with car accidents; *ergo*, let us ban cars and there will be no more car accidents," may be relevant for public health, but it is not science.

Black box epidemiology disparages understanding. It takes short-cuts to be able to issue "warnings," which, because of the nature of studied "exposures," often overlap with exhortations of politically correct moralists. Epidemiologists from Utah warned that "passive" smoking is a risk factor for cervical cancer, and of the same magnitude as that of active smoking. They defended this absurd claim as follows: "While we do not know of a biological mechanism for either active or passive smoking to be related to cervical cancer, we do know that cigarette smoking is harmful to health. The message to the public, as a result of this study, is one that reinforces the message that smoking is detrimental to health."[7]

The futility of black box research can be demonstrated by the example of the endless stream of studies attempting to implicate coffee drinking as the "cause" of various diseases. As the United States imports some 3 billion pounds of coffee annually, its ubiquitous consumption might have been of public health importance, if and only if there were a shred of evidence that the various associations reported in the epidemiologic literature are truly causal. For the past 30 years, a debate has been going on whether coffee drinking is causally linked to coronary heart disease. Three different positions have been taken: the risk of coronary heart disease in coffee drinkers is increased, not changed, or decreased. The impasse is unlikely to he resolved by further case-control studies. The same can be said about the associations between coffee drinking and bladder cancer: a recent review of 35 case-control studies, spanning 20 years of wasted effort, failed to find any clinically important association.[8] These are examples of the mindless repetition of black box research, which, far from being "stabs in the dark," is more like the repetitive punching of a well-lit soft pillow; when the dimple refills, it is ready for another blow. More adventurous risk factor epidemiologists have studied associations between coffee drinking and cancers of pancreas, breast, colon, rectum, and ovary. Others discovered a "clear protective effect" against colonic adenomas in drinkers of more than eight cups of coffee a day [odds ratio (OR) = 0.3; 95% confidence interval (CI) = 0.1-0.6].[9] Data dredging from the Framingham study led to a report that coffee (or tea) drinking is a risk factor for hip fractures.[10] As Feinstein and his colleagues[11] have pointed out, the credibility of risk factor epidemiology can withstand only a limited number of false alarms.

An area in which Savitz has a special interest, the associations of electromagnetic field exposures and cancer, is another example of a soft pillow that refills each time it is punched. As noted by the Oak Ridge Associated Universities (ORAU) Panel on Health Effects of Low-Frequency Electric and Magnetic Fields, three recent Swedish studies produced mutually exclusive results.[12] For childhood leukemia, one study found a positive association, whereas another reported a negative association. For adult brain tumors, one study showed an increased risk, whereas another study found a declining trend. For adult lymphatic leukemia, the risk increased in one study but appeared to decrease in another study. In one of the studies, in which magnetic fields were actually measured, rather than estimated, no positive association was found with any malignancies. The link between electromagnetic fields and cancer is not only empirically weak or irreproducible, but it is also biologically implausible. Electrical fields generated at the surface of the brain or heart are comparable in strength with those induced on the body surface by nearby power lines, and even an ordinary stroll, at a speed of 1 meter per second, in the earth's geomagnetic field induces greater electrical fields in the body of the walker than magnetic fields from overhead power lines.

Black box epidemiology is not science: it resembles the futile search for a *perpetuum mobile*. Even if reported associations were real, rather than spurious, the black box approach can be compared with the reaction of a TV watcher who does not like a particular programme. He does not care what happens in the "black box" (that is, the TV set), but he knows that he can stop the programme by switching off the power. Even in this comparison, risk factor epidemiology is at a disadvantage, since it does not know the location of the "switch," nor whether the "switch" functions as a switch. A better analogy might be the association between suicide by hanging and the availability of rope. It does not follow that the removal of ropes would eliminate suicides by hanging (what about shoelaces, etc?). Even if all ropes and all rope analogues were banned, it still does not follow that the incidence of suicide would decline. To understand the phenomenon of suicide, it is essential to open the "black box" of psychological processes that lead to the decision to take one's own life. To calculate the relative risk of suicide among the owners of firearms is neither psychology nor science. An example of such nonsense calculation comes from an abstract of a report presented at the annual meeting of the Society for Epidemiological Research, with the title "Case-Control Study of Which Dogs Bite."[13] Odds ratios for biting a "non-household member" were increased for German shepherds and chows, but also for dogs residing in a house with one or more children (OR = 3.5; 95% CI = 1.6-7.5). This odds ratio was higher than for unneutered dogs (OR = 2.6) or for dogs chained in the yard (OR = 2.8). The author concluded, with a logical *non sequitur*, that people may "modify the risk by neutering dogs and not keeping them chained," without suggesting, by dint of the same logic, that they should have less than one child.

Savitz is right to conclude that there is no logical link between the quality of epidemiologic studies and the state of knowledge in other disciplines. I am not aware that anyone ever suggested that such a link exists. By the same token, there is no logical link between black box epidemiologic studies and science. Savitz, however, is wrong in suggesting that "[v]alid epidemiologic studies contribute to science and public health whether we ignore, build upon, or contradict parallel information derived from other disciplines." Risk factor epidemiology is an ancillary methodology, which, if governed by rigorous scientific principles may provide testable hypotheses of causality. It cannot "contradict" pertinent scientific data, and it ignores them only at its peril.

References

1. Savitz DA. In defense of black box epidemiology.
   Epidemiology 1994; 5: 553-555
2. Doll R, Peto R. The causes of cancer: quantitative estimates of avoidable risks of cancer in the United States today.
   J Natl Cancer Inst 1981;66:1191-1305.
3. Thomas L. An epidemic of apprehension.
   Discover 1983; November: 78-79.
4. Feinstein A. Scientific standards in epidemiological studies of the menaces of daily life. *Science* 1988; 242: 1257-1263.
5. Vandenbroucke JP. Is "the causes of cancer" a miasma theory for the end of the twentieth century?
   Int J Epidemiol 1988; 17: 708-709.
6. Skrabanek P. Risk factor epidemiology: science or non-science? In Health, Lifestyle and Environment: Countering the Panic. Manhattan Institute, New York, 1991: 47-56.
7. Slattery ML Exposure to cigarette smoke and cervical cancer.
   JAMA 1989; 262: 499
8. Viscoli CM, Lachs MS, Horwitz RI. Bladder cancer and coffee drinking: a summary of case-control research. *Lancet* 1993; 341:
9. Olsen J, Kronborg O. Coffee, tobacco and alcohol as risk factors for cancer and adenoma of the large intestine.
   Int J Epidemiol 1993; 22: 398-402.
10. Kiel DP, Felson DT, Hannan MT, Anderson JJ, Wilson PWF. Caffeine and the risk of hip fracture: the Framingham study.
    Am J Epidemiol 1990; 132: 675-684.

11. Feinstein AR, Horowitz RI, Spitzer WO, Battista RN. Coffee and pancreatic cancer: the problem of etiologic science and epidemiological case-control research. *JAMA* 1981; 246: 957-961.
12. ORAU Panel on Health Effects of Low-Frequency Electric and Magnetic Fields. EMF and cancer. *Science* 1993: 260: 13-14.
13. Gershman K.Case-control study of which dogs bite (Abstract). *Am J Epidemiol* 1993; 138: 593.

15

IRISH TRADITIONAL MEDICINE: THE FOXGLOVE ORDEAL AND OTHER FOLK 'CURES'

In Ireland, much of folk medicine has been quietly forgotten and gradually replaced by the foreign import of 'alternative' medicine, in its endless variations. Gone are most bone-setters, herbalists, fairy doctors, wise women and hedge practitioners. Their place has been taken by 'counsellors' and smartly dressed entrepreneurs, with strings of idiosyncratic degrees behind their names, and with surgeries on the main street or in shopping plazas. Spinologists, aromatherapists, experts in Chinese or Indian medicines, self-realisation therapists, rebirthers and karma-clearers, educational kinesiologists, reflexologists, iridologists, acupuncturists...

Folk medicine should not be confused with primitive medicine, since in addition to true primitive traits it contains degenerate high cultural elements.[1] Primitive medicine is the precursor of folk medicine, alternative medicine and rational medicine. Alternative medicine is akin to folk medicine in its mixture of magic and modern cultural elements, but it differs from it in its need for systematisation and rationalisation imitating science. Not all 'orthodox' medicine is rational either. Furthermore, the false glitter of alternative medicine has irresistible appeal even for some ordinary doctors, who, disillusioned with the slow progress of rational medicine and untrained in critical thinking, embrace new panaceas as their predecessors did in the past.

The handful of traditional folk healers still surviving in Ireland were divided by the folklorist Buckley into three groups: (1) those on whom a 'cure' was passed on as a hereditary right; (2) those who acquire a cure by being the seventh son (or daughter), or a posthumous child, or a

---

This paper first appeared in the *Journal of the Irish Colleges of Physicians and Surgeons* 1994; Vol 23 No 2: pages 121-126. Reproduced by kind permission.

Irish traditional medicine

woman who marries a husband with the same surname; and (3) faith healers who discover their ability to heal within themselves.[2]

The passed-on cures and the acquired cures are often limited to a single condition, such as whooping cough, ringworm, or cancer. The passed-on cures are generally some magic formula for an ointment or a 'plaster'; their composition is kept secret, and they are effective only when accompanied by a silent prayer known only to the healer. The acquired cures are no trade secrets. They may amount to no more than offering the patient (with the specific condition) a cup of tea, a piece of bread, or a ritual combination of three liquids, such as tea, milk, and lemonade. Buckley describes the predicament of women who marry someone with the same name. Within a few weeks of their marriage, someone may knock on the door saying, 'I hear you have the cure for whooping cough.' If the woman does not know what to do, the mother of the sick child may instruct her in the proper ritual. In the case of seventh sons (about whom more later), some may stick to the traditional cure of ringworm, or farcy in horses, but many become faith healers.

Much of folk medicine is of a do-it-yourself nature, whether for benign, self-limiting conditions, such as the dozens of recommendations for the disappearance of warts, or for more serious ailments, pilgrimage to holy wells. Many primitive cures, still practised within the past 100 years, have their parallels in other parts of the world, such as the healing power of fasting spittle, drinking one's own urine, or dosing children with cow urine, application of cow dung on cuts and wounds, the use of red flannel for various ailments, or tea made of sheep's droppings for measles. Some are more indigenous, such as snuff left over from a wake as a cure for headache, or carrying a potato in the pocket as a prophylactic against rheumatism.

Magical thinking is not limited to the simple folk. Until the 19th century, treatment of disease described in medical textbooks was no more rational than the magic of folk healers.

Tar water

The most famous Irish philosopher, Bishop Berkeley (1685-1753) was described by T.E. Jessop, an authority on Berkeley, as having 'an irresistible itch to clarify thinking', and yet when it came to disease and health, his mind became hopelessly befuddled. He convinced himself that tar water was the nearest natural thing to drinkable God,[3] a universal panacea and the ultimate life-preservative. In his tract *Siris, A Chain of Philosophical Reflections and Inquiries concerning the Virtue of Tar Water* (1744) Berkeley, carried away by his discovery, wrote: 'I freely own that I suspect Tar-water is a panacea ... If I had a situation high enough, and the voice loud enough, I would cry out to all valetudinarians upon Earth, drink Tar water'.[4]

The unquestioning simplicity of a folk healer differs little from the learned naiveté of philosophers, priests and doctors of the past.

Foxglove

It is commonly believed that herbalists sit on a treasure-house of cures, discovered by patient empirical observation over the centuries. The idea that herbal lore is based on empiricism betrays a misunderstanding of its magical origin and nature, and is an example of rationalising irrational attempts, over centuries, to change the natural course of sickness. While the immense plant kingdom is a veritable laboratory in which an enormous array of wonderful chemicals are effortlessly produced, it does not follow that for each disease there exists a plant which would cure it. Only a handful of useful remedies have been derived from plants. Much more interesting is the use of euphoriant or hallucinogenic plants in all cultures and its suppression by authority, simply because people find the experience pleasurable.

One of the few plants always invoked when the value of herbalism is questioned is foxglove. Its Latin name *Digitalis* was bestowed upon it by the German botanist Leonhard Fuchs in 1542. (His name is immortalised in fuchsia, whose bushes with their blood-red flowers adorn the hedges of Irish boreens.) Foxglove is mentioned in medieval herbals, its use mainly as an emetic and purgative. Its diuretic properties were first described by William Withering in 1785, following ten years of careful observation on 167 patients.[5] His interest was first aroused by a local 'cure' for dropsy, which was a herbal tea made of some twenty plants. He recognised the foxglove as the important constituent. Within 15 years of the publication of his observations, digitalis became another panacea, used mainly for conditions in which it could do no good.

A poor understanding of human pathophysiology precluded even the medical profession from using digitalis rationally. It took another 100 years after Withering's Account to change 'dropsy' from a disease to a nonspecific sign. Herbalists fared no better. According to Logan, who was collecting Irish herb-lore for 30 years, foxglove was never used for any heart condition.[6]

When Moloney surveyed the herbal uses for his Pioneering publication *Luibh-Sheanchus, Irish Ethno-Botany and the Evolution of Medicine in Ireland* (1919), his informants denied that foxglove was ever used internally, though one person had heard of its use in ointments for 'scrophulous swellings', that is, the King's evil.[7]

In an Irish herbal from 1735 by John K'Eogh (*Botanalogia Universalis Hibernica, or, A General Irish Herbal, Calculated for this Kingdom, giving an Account of the Herbs, Shrubs, and Trees, naturally produced therein, in English, Irish, and Latin, &c.*), the indications for foxglove are given as follows: 'The decoction of it drank dissolves viscous and slimy humours. It opens opulations of the liver and spleen. It is a great catharctic and emetic, working violently upwards and downwards. It is good for any obstruction of the lungs, as also for the epilepsy. An ointment made of it is exceedingly good for all scrophulous ulcers. Made into a poultis, with hogs-lard, cures the Kings-Evil, drinking the juice of water parsnip in clarified cheese whey'.[8]

The most common indication for the use of foxglove was a charm against witchcraft. Lady Wilde, the mother of Oscar Wilde, in her *Ancient Cures, Charms, and Usages of Ireland* (1890) records, rather cryptically, that 'a bewitched person may die under the treatment (with foxglove), especially if tied naked to a stake, as was the custom in old times, while the imprecation is said, if you are bewitched, or fairy-struck, may the devil take you away, with the curse on your head for ever and ever'.[9]

The nature of these ordeals in the 19th century was described by Dr. William Pickells, from the Fever Hospital in Cork, who in 1828 commented on a widespread superstition 'among the lower orders' in his part of the country, who believed or pretended to believe that 'children labouring under consumptive, ricketty, or other cachectic and wasting diseases' were changelings, that is, substituted by fairies who stole the real child. Such children were given a foxglove brew to drink, in the belief that if the child dies it was not a human being, as foxglove was said to be poisonous only to fairies. Pickells suspected, rightly it would seem, that this trial by foxglove was a socially sanctioned form of infanticide. He knew of many such cases.[10] In March 1851, a woman named Bridget Peters, 'a fairy doctress' was convicted at the Assizes at Nenagh of killing a child with foxglove. The child, about 6 years old had some kind of paralysis and the treatment consisted of dosing it repeatedly with foxglove and exposing it at night on a shovel on a dunghill, where it was found one day dead.[10]

An anonymous correspondent to the *Lancet* (Oct 15, 1831) signing himself as 'a medical student', provided further details of this practice in Ireland. In the case of children with epilepsy - a disease thought to be symptomatic of the child being a changeling, or 'fairy-stricken' - the child was 'challenged' (to use the modern medical term) with foxglove: 'A consultation of old women is held, with a *ban lieughth*' * or a woman skilled with herbs, as president. The fairy is counselled to leave the house quietly, and send back the people's child. If he continue obstinate, they first threaten him with... (sitting him) on a red-hot shovel or roasting him at the fire. These threats being disregarded and the fairy's presence being still ascertained by the recurrence of the fits, he is at last doomed to take the digitalis, a dose considered most obnoxious to the fairy tribe'.[11]

Pickells reports another case from an inquest held in the county Tipperary in April 1840. A child, named John Mahony, aged 6 to 7,

---

ban-liaigh (woman-leech; fairy doctress) or possibly *bean luibhe* (woman of herbs) was confined to bed for two years 'with affection of the spine' and the parents thought he was a changeling. He was threatened in the usual way with a red-hot shovel and with ducking under a pump, until he finally 'confessed' that he was a fairy. On the following day he was found dead.

Hydrophobia

As for any incurable disease, cures and charms against hydrophobia abounded. The distinction should be made, however, between the bite of a 'mad' dog (which was not necessarily a rabid dog) and rabies.

Lady Wilde in her *Ancient Cures* mentions that 'in old times, in Ireland, people afflicted with canine madness were put to death by smothering between two feather beds; the near relatives standing round until asphyxia was produced and death followed'.[9] This form of euthanasia was not restricted to Ireland only, as a similar practice existed in Brittany and in other parts of France.[12]

Another such case was recalled by an informant from Ulster, whose father remembered how a young boy, bitten by a mad dog, developed hydrophobia and 'the father and an uncle smothered the child between two ticks, feather ticks, and apparently there was no law to prevent that'.[13]

These acts of desperation, tempered by mercy, are probably more understandable to ordinary people than to theologians. Peasants would kill injured animals to 'put them out of misery', and the same compassion was extended, in extreme circumstances, to their own kin. Both Partridge and Ballard suggested that the practice was probably widespread.[12,13]

Abortifacients

Desmond Corrigan, from the Dept. of Pharmacognosy, TCD, reviewed the state of folk herbal medicine in Ireland in a lecture he gave at a joint conference of the Botanical Society and the Folklore Society, in 1983, and suggested that 'there are no records of plants with abortifacient or contraceptive uses', which he thought was 'not surprising, given the religious nature of Irish people'.[14]

If this were true, Ireland would be a world exception, since abortion of unwanted pregnancies has been attempted by women in all societies and at all times, regardless of the prevailing religious ideology or severe penalties. More likely, in a climate where abortion is still seen as an abomination, informants would be more than reluctant to own up to such knowledge or practice.

The earliest record of a pregnancy termination in Ireland comes, curiously, from Life of St Brigid the Virgin, written by Cogitosus in the 7th Century: 'A certain woman who had taken the vow of chastity fell, through youthful desire of pleasure, and her womb swelled with child. Brigid, exercising the most potent strength of her ineffable faith, blessed her, causing the foetus to disappear, without coming to birth, and without pain'.[15]

John K'Eogh, who was chaplain to Lord Kingston in Cork, lists in his *Botanalogia Universalis Hibernica*,[8] a large number of plants described as 'emmenagogues', or capable of 'expelling the dead child', or being 'very hurtful to woman with child' (e.g. honeysuckle), or very dangerous for women with child to make use of it, or to step over it' (sow-bread, *Cyclamen*). This preoccupation with missed periods in the eighteenth-century Ireland would suggest that unwanted pregnancy was as much a worry then as it is today. What is ironic, and perhaps disturbing, is that an edited version of this herbal, 'rendered suitable for the modern reader', is on sale in Dublin as a 'practical handbook', according to the publisher's announcement on the back cover.

When on the subject of fertility and its antidotes, it is amusing to note that K'Eogh classified potato as 'spermatogenic'.

Henry Purdon, physician to Belfast Skin Hospital, listed various popular Irish herb remedies and noted that in 1895 there was still one herbalist selling his wares at the Belfast Vegetable Market.[16] On the stall, Purdon saw tansy (*Tanacetum vulgare*), which was then considered 'an emmenagogue of much power', and he mentioned another local plant, centaury (*Erythraea pulchella*), which, according to Culpepper's Herbal of 1653 is useful for bringing on the 'courses in women, helps to void the dead-birth and eases the mother's pains'.

Moloney in his *Irish Ethno-Botany* (1919) is more reticent in mentioning such uses. He reports that garden marigold (*Calendula officinalis*) is recommended as a 'uterine tonic', and that shepherd's purse (*Capsella bursa pastoris*) was used as 'emmenagogue'.[7]

King's Evil

Foxglove was only one of the plants recommended for the cure of 'scrofula'. In Ireland, some herbalists used shamrock for the same purpose. John Knott, a Trinity graduate and an authority on Irish folklore, befriended a Co. Roscommon man whose only link with the healing profession was 'by forming the last link of the chain — in the capacity of grave-digger'. The sexton's cure for the 'running evil', as he called it, was a poultice made from the leaves of the cuckoo-sorrel, followed by a dressing made of the root of the sweet-meadow.[17] The cuckoo-sorrel, also known as wood sorrel (*Oxalis acetosella*) was thought by several authorities to be the original Irish shamrock, since wood sorrel was 'the only green thing which could be found on the first of March' and since, as reported by travellers from the 16th century, the Irish used shamrock for food and it had a sharp, sour taste.[18] The commercial shamrock is grown from seed of the yellow clover (*Trifolium dubium*) and the earliest written mention of the practice of wearing a trefoil in commemoration of St. Patrick appears only in 1726, when the white clover (*Trifolium repens*) was indicated.[18] However, in a 1988 survey, there was still a small minority of respondents who claimed that wood sorrel was the true 'dear little, sweet little shamrock of Ireland'.[19]

Knott found references to the wood sorrel in many old herbals, for example in the Parkinson's *Theatrum Botanicum* (1640), where it is recommended for 'any hot tumours and inflammations which it does exceedingly coole and helpe them'.[17] K'eogh described the wood sorrel as 'cordial, stomatic, hepatic and hydrotic, good against the jaundice and dropsy. It also modified and heals rotten ulcers'.[8] In Wicklow, at the beginning of this century, the wood sorrel was still a panacea: 'any badness that would be in the system it would drive it out'.[20]

King's Evil, or 'scrophula' was not a single disease. Any swelling, be it

Irish traditional medicine

goitre, boil, tumour or tuberculous scrofula, or any ulcerating lesion, not necessarily on the neck, would qualify. Knott pointed out that the cures for the King's Evil and for the French pox were often identical. Eminent physicians had their favourite prescription for this disease, ranging from oil made from boiling frogs to rubbing the sore with a dead man's hand. The latter cure was recommended for example by the celebrated Thomas Bartholinus.[17]

In England (and also in France), kings, and sometimes queens, were endowed with the miraculous gift of curing the King's Evil (*mal de roi*) by touch.[21] In Ireland, the King being inaccessible on account of the distance, the royal treatment had to be by proxy. A woman in Co. Roscommon, known to Knott, used to treat the King's Evil by touching the sores with a linen rag which contained the 'royal blood and remains'.[17] Dr. Marlay Blake recalled, in a lecture he gave in Dundalk in 1917, that for generations his family was credited with the ability to cure King's Evil by means of a thread from a handkerchief once dipped in the blood of Charles I. He also mentioned that his great uncle, Walter Blake, suspected of suffering from rabies. met his death by being smothered between featherbeds.[22]

The belief in the healing touch of a dead man's hand has survived in Ireland to this century. For example, people in Wicklow believed that the touch of a dead man's hand would cure a birth mark.[20] One folklorist reported the following cure from Donegal in 1912. Her informant's father died and her neighbour woman came in and said: 'Will you be pleased to lift your father's hand, an' rub it on this sore arm o' mine? I dinna like to do it mysel'. Then she rolled up her sleeve and exposed a big lump on her arm, addressing the corpse, 'Take my pains wi' you, Mick, for the love of God!'[23]

This superstition is of old vintage. In Pliny's *Historiae naturalis*, Book xxviii, par. 11, we are assured that 'the hand of a person carried off by premature death cures by a touch scrofulous sores, diseased parotid glands, and throat affections; some however say that the back of any dead person's left hand will do this if the patient is of the same sex'.[24]

While English and French monarchs had to use their royal hands for curing their subjects, King Pyrrhus (c. 318-272 B.C.) achieved the same results by using the great toe of his right foot, as again Pliny assures us. This method has survived in Ireland to this day. The folklorist Buckley discovered an Irish seventh daughter, whose curative technique involves placing her bare foot on the patient's back.[2] Is this a pyrrhic victory for unreason, or just the result of democratisation and of the end of sex discrimination?

Laying-on of hands

During his 25-year reign, Charles II was said to have touched up to 100,000 sick persons. But many lay competitors, usurping the royal prerogative, tried their hands at it. The most famous Irish 'stroker', as they were known, was Valentine Greatrakes (1629-1683). He was Clerk of Peace for the County of Cork and Registrar of Transplantation, in which capacity he was recording the export of Irish women and children as slaves to the West Indies. Greatrakes discovered his miraculous ability to heal by touch when he was made unemployed with the departure of Cromwell from Ireland. Feeling dejected he was brooding over his predicament until one day when he announced to his wife that God bestowed on him the gift of curing the King's Evil. His wife, being a sensible woman, dismissed this politely as a 'strange imagination', but patients started flocking to his door from far and wide. He won the confidence of the scientist Robert Boyle, himself the seventh son of the Earl of Cork, and of other luminaries in the world of science, philosophy and theology. He became a darling of aristocracy. "Lady Ranelagh frequently amused the guests at her routs with Mr. Valentine Greatrakes, who in the character of the lion of the season performed with wondrous results on the prettiest or most hysterical of the ladies present."[17] His urine was said to smell of violets.[25]

The Protestant Greatrakes sprang to fame when James Finaghty, a Catholic priest and exorcist, sank into obscurity. Finaghty also used stroking, besides prayer and 'blowing vehemently into the ears of the diseased party'.[26] As More Madden, obstetrician in the Mater Misericordiae Hospital in Dublin, noted, 'the practice of blowing into the ears of cattle, especially horses, was old popular arcanum well known to cattle doctors and veterinary practitioners in this country.'[26] Finaghty had charge of a parish in the Archbishopric of Tuam, but according to a letter from an Irish Jesuit, quoted by Madden, Finaghty was raised up by Providence in the time of trouble to confirm the people in their religion, and he drew thousands, 'who followed him even through bogs, woods, mountains and rocks, and desert places, whithersoever the people heard him to have fled from the persecution of Cromwell's officers and governors, that priests enough could not be had (though many accompanied him on purpose) to hear the Confessions of the great multitude drawn to repentance and resolutions of a new life by the example of his life and wonder of his works, that, therefore, he was esteemed a Thaumaturgus, or wonder-worker of Ireland.'

The current fashion of healing by the laying on of hands began with American and European faith healers in the last century. In Ireland, as in Central and Western Europe, an older tradition exists, according to which the seventh son has a magical (non-religious) power to heal by touch. Being born as the seventh son (without interpolated daughters) is not as unlikely as it may seem. The probability is 1:128, and families with 7 children were by no means uncommon. In Biscay and Catalonia, seventh sons were credited with the power to cure rabies, while in France or Great Britain they were good at curing scrofula. The Irish seventh sons were traditionally curers of ringworm.[21] Seventh daughters were ignored, but according to one Irish commentator, the seventh daughter of a seventh daughter should be given wide berth as such oddities had an evil eye.[27]

The belief in the magic of the seventh son is still current in Ireland. Some of them advertise in Old Moore's Almanac. For example in the 1991 Almanac (page 69), John Doran, 'internationally known 7th son of a 7th son faith healer' asks 'Have you a health problem that you cannot get help with? Have you a family worry that you need advice about? Absent healing a specially. Future trends also given. Call, write or phone' with a telephone number and address.

One such healer was profiled in the Irish Times recently (Jan 19, 1993).

Irish traditional medicine

He was a hospital security guard until he was thrown off his motorbike and experienced a vision of 'Our Lady the Virgin Mary floating in mid-air, about three feet from the ground'. The day after the accident his hands started bleeding, which he attributed to stigmatisation. Soon after he discovered that he acquired the ability of curing AIDS, cancer, deafness, blindness, brain tumours and Parkinsonism. By coincidence, he happened also to be a seventh son.

The best known Irish seventh son is Finbarr Nolan. His healing powers were discovered when he was two years old. Following a T.V. programme about him in 1970, when he was 17, hundreds of sick people were queuing at his doorstep. Within a year he bought his first Jaguar XJ6. 'I believe I was the youngest person in the world at that time driving around in a Jaguar bought by myself from my own money', he writes in his autobiography.[28] In his book he claims cures of multiple sclerosis, cancer, blindness, deafness, epilepsy, tuberculosis and AIDS. Once he even cured a dog of cancer, he writes. His healing circuit now includes also Britain and the USA.

While seventh sons get their gifts through the power vested in the number seven, other healers obtain their ability to cure the incurable by a spiritual effort. On June 13, 1990 the *Irish Times* carried a feature on a 'very Christian orientated couple, Peter and Elisabeth Gill', who practise spiritual healing. In their house in Co. Wicklow, there is a room called the 'Colour Light Sanctuary, a little room in which Peter (an engineer retired from the motor industry) has introduced a lighting system which at a touch of a switch can provide whichever colour is best suited to your form of healing. On a table in the centre lie dozens of opened letters, petitions for 'absent healing' or 'distant healing', written on behalf of those who are either unwilling or unable to receive 'contact' healing'.

'Distant healing' is also advocated by the President of the Irish Association of Holistic Medicine, Mr. Martin Forde, who runs various courses in the Tony Quinn Organisation in Dublin. In their newsletter, which is dropped into the letterboxes of 500,000 households, according to its own advertisement, the readers have been invited to fill in a coupon with a 'request' either for themselves or on behalf of friends or relatives. From letters by satisfied customers, printed in this newsletter, it is made clear that readers can request not only a distant cure but also the fulfilment of their wish, such as getting a job, or a new car, or passing an exam. It costs merely £20 a month per one request.

References

1. Ackerknecht EH. Problems of primitive medicine. *Bull Hist Med* 1942; 11: 503-521.

2. Buckley AD. Unofficial healing in Ulster. *Ulster Folklife* 1980; 26: 15-34..

3. Berman D. Bishop Berkeley and the fountains of living waters. *Hermathena* 1980; 128: 21-31.

4. Berkeley G. Siris, a chain of philosophical reflections and inquiries concerning the virtue of tar water. 2nd ed. Dublin, 1744.

5. Withering W. An account of the foxglove and some of its uses. with practical remarks on dropsy, and other diseases. M. Swinney, Birmingham, 1785.

6. Logan P. Making the cure. A look at Irish folk medicine. Talbot Press, Dublin, 1972.

7. Moloney MF. Luibh-sheanchus. Irish ethno-botany and the evolution of medicine in Ireland. M.H. Gill & Son, Dublin, 1919.

8. K'Eogh J. Botanalogia univeralis Hibernica, or, A general Irish herbal, calculated for this kingdom, giving an account of the herbs, shrubs, and trees, naturally produced therein, in English, Irish, and Latin; with a true description of them, and their medicinal virtues and qualities, etc. G. Harrison, Corke, 1735.

9. Lady Wilde. Ancient cures, charms, and usages of Ireland. Contributions to Irish lore. Waed & Downey, London, 1890.

10. Pickells W. Deleterius practice of some of the Irish peasantry connected with the belief in fairies. *Edinburgh Med Surg J* 1851; 76:57-63.

11 Anon. Digitalis In epilepsy. *Lancet* 1831/1832; i: 98.

12 Partridge A. A traditional method of dealing with rabies victims. *Béaloideas* 1980; 48/49: 204-205.

13 Ballard L-M. Traditional treatment of hydrophobia. Ulster Folklife 1986; 32: 83-86.

14 Corrigan D. The scientific basis of folk medicine: the Irish dimension. In: Vickery R.ed. Plant-lore studies. The Folklore Society, London, 1984: 1042.

15 De Paor L. St. Patrick's world. Christian culture of Ireland's apostolic age. Four Courts, Dublin, 1993.

16 Purdon HS Notes on old native remedies. *Dublin J Med Sci* 1895; 100: 214-218, 293-296.

17 Knott J. A country herbalist's cure for the King's Evil. *Med Press* 1899; 119:1-4, 32-34, 56-57, 80-82, 108-110, 132-134, 157-159.

18 Frazer W. The shamrock; its history. *J Roy Soc Antiquaries Ireland* 1894; 24: 132-135.

19 Nelson EC. Shamrock 1988. *Ulster Folklife* 1990; 36: 32-42.

20 Ó Cléirigh T. Gleanings in Co. Wicklow. *Béaloideas* 1928; 1: 245-252.

21 Bloch M. The royal touch: sacred monarchy and scrofula in England and France. Routledge & Kegan Paul, London, 1973.

22 Blake RM. Folk lore. With some account of the ancient Gaelic leeches and the state of art of medicine in ancient Erin. *J Co Louth Archaeol Soc* 1918; 4: 217-225.

23 M'Clintock L. Donegal cures and charms. *Folk-Lore* 1912; 23: 473-478.

24 Pliny. Natural history, vol. 8. Translated by Jones WHS. Heinemann, London, 1963.

25 Thomas K. Religion and the decline of magic. Studies in popular beliefs in sixteenth- and seventeenth-century England. Penguin, Harmondsworth, 1973.

26 Madden TM. On the recent revival, under new names, of some old fallacies bearing on medicine. *Dublin J Med Sci* 1890; 90: 22-41.

27 Fleming JB. Folklore, fact and legend. *Ir J Med Sci* 1953; 6th Ser, No. 326:49-63.

28 Nolan F. (with Duffy M.). Seventh son of a seventh son. The life story of a healer. Mainstream Publishing, Edinburgh, 1992.

16

A SUBVERSIVE MAN

Richard Feynman, who died on Feb 15, 1988, at the age of 69, was probably the only man who, on July 16, 1945, actually saw the explosion of the first atomic bomb. "They gave out dark glasses that you could watch it with. Dark glasses! Twenty miles away, you couldn't see a damn thing through dark glasses! I figured that the only thing that could hurt your eyes is ultraviolet light. I got behind a truck windshield, because the ultraviolet light can't go through glass, so that would be safe and so I could see the damn thing."

When Princeton physicists were recruited *en bloc* for the Manhattan Project, they were instructed not to buy train tickets from Princeton in order not to create suspicion that something was up. Feynman, reasoning that if everybody bought their tickets somewhere else . . . , bought his at the Princeton station. Only then did the station-master think he understood for whom were all those crates shipped for weeks from Princeton to Albuquerque — Mr Feynman was moving! When working on the bomb, Feynman developed an interest in the combination locks guarding top-secret materials, and was soon able to open them all. Instead of getting better locks, they kept Feynman away from them.

The two books of Feynman's memoirs, as recorded by Ralph Leighton (a son of Feynman's fellow professor at the California Institute of Technology and a drumming partner in a group called The Three Quarks),[1,2] present, in the words of a fellow physicist Freeman Dyson, a "wise, funny, simple, profound, cool, passionate and totally honest self-portrait" of one of the most extraordinary characters and one of the greatest theoretical physicists.

This paper first appeared in *The Lancet* 1989; i: 94-95
© The Lancet Ltd. Reproduced by kind permission of The Lancet Ltd.

A subversive man

Feynman seemed to cherish his acceptance as a *frigideira* player by a Brazilian samba band during his sabbatical at the University of Rio more than the Nobel Prize he won in 1965 for "the fundamental work in quantum electrodynamics with deep-ploughing consequences for the physics of elementary particles". Among his other contributions, he worked out, with a fellow eccentric, Murray Gell-Mann, the theory of ß-decay. (Gell-Mann, who got his Nobel Prize four years later, is an accomplished linguist and a student of *Finnegans Wake*; for his theory of quarks he found the term "quark" on the first line of book ii, chapter 4 of *Finnegans Wake*. People used to say that Caltech appointed Gell-Mann so that Feynman would have someone to talk to.) Feynman, on the other hand, learnt Japanese and gave public lectures on Mayan hieroglyphics. Hans Bethe recalled how Feynman once taught two classes simultaneously, standing in the doorway and writing diagrams of nuclear fission on two blackboards at the same time with both hands.

Accounts of liaisons with bar girls in nightclubs and casinos (with asides on the mathematics of gambling) alternate with stories about the joy of doing and teaching physics, playing bongo drums, drawing nude models and being commissioned to paint a nude female torreador for a massage parlour, encounters with pompous fools and royalty, having a sniffing competition with his own dog, and corruption in school-book publishing. A hilarious story which tells how Feynman was declared unfit for military service by army psychiatrists is a classic which could have come from the pen of Leacock or Twain. Once he agreed to testify in a court case that topless bars were acceptable to the Pasadena community. He did this as a favour to a proprietor of one such establishment in which he used to write up his lectures. "The Caltech professor of physics goes to see topless dancing six times a week", ran a newspaper headline. What these memoirs breathe with is the sheer fun of life and of intellectual enjoyment, conveying at the same time the unquenchable thirst of a beautiful mind for understanding.

When Feynman was asked to join the commission of inquiry into the

Challenger shuttle disaster, his first reaction was not to go anywhere near Washington ("screw the Government") and to continue doing his physics for as long as his abdominal cancer would allow him. When he finally accepted he became a legend overnight when, in front of TV cameras, he dropped a piece of a rubber ring (which was to seal the booster rocket but did not) into ice-water and demonstrated how the rubber lost its resilience. In his minority report, published, after attempts to stall it failed, as an appendix F to the main report, Feynman accused NASA of playing Russian roulette with the lives of the crew, and concluded that "a successful technology must take precedence over public relations, for Nature cannot be fooled". The bulk of the second memoir[2] is an inimitable account of Feynman's own investigations into the cause and the background of the catastrophe.

Feynman's scientific credo was encapsulated in two public lectures — on Cargo Cult Science and on the Value of Science. This belies the "powerful sense of social irresponsibility" of which Feynman liked to boast. Pseudoscience (in which Feynman includes educational theories, parapsychology, and much of medicine) is like cargo-cult rituals in the South Seas. During the war the islanders had seen aeroplanes landing with lots of goods and they imagined that, if they built airstrips, lit fires along them, and sat a man in a hut, as a controller, with two pieces of wood for headphones and some bamboo sticks for aerials, planes would bring cargoes of goodies again. The form is the same but it does not work — no planes land. There is nothing easier than fooling ourselves and others. Schools provide no courses in self-defence against wishful thinking. Feynman insisted on scrupulous honesty in presenting *all* data from experiments, on bending over backwards to show we may have been wrong — this he saw as the scientist's main responsibility. Above all he defended the need for complete freedom of inquiry. "In order to progress we must recognise our ignorance and leave room for doubt ... our freedom to doubt was born out of a struggle against authority ... permit us to question, to doubt, not to be sure ... Herein lies a responsibility to society ... It is our responsibility as scientists, knowing the great progress which comes from a satisfactory philosophy of ignorance, the great progress which is the fruits of freedom of thought, to proclaim the value of this freedom, to teach how doubt is not to be feared but welcomed and discussed, and to demand this freedom as our duty to all coming generations."

Amidst the aggravating madness of this absurd world, these words give a glimmer of hope. I even feel proud of being human because Feynman existed. Every teacher and every student should read these two books: the teachers to examine their consciences and to reflect on how they have been enslaving young minds; the students to learn how to recover their natural subversiveness and to rediscover the joy of free inquiry.

References

1. Feynman RP. Surely, you're joking, Mr. Feynman! Adventures of a curious character. Unwin Paperbacks, London, 1986.
2. Feynman RP. What do you care what other people think? Further adventures of a curious character. Unwin Hyman, London, 1989.